C. Nickl-Weller | S. Matthys | T. Eichenauer | C. Wagenaar (Eds.)

Fast & Flexible

Medizinisch Wissenschaftliche Verlagsgesellschaft

C. Nickl-Weller | S. Matthys | T. Eichenauer | C. Wagenaar (Eds.)

Fast & Flexible

Planning for Adaptive Health Care Systems

Health Care of the Future 9

Contributors:
M. Barrett | J. Brunet | J.F. Debatin | M. Di Marco | L. Fontana
A. Gebhard | R. de Graaf | F. Jensen | C. Lohfert Praetorius
S. Matthys | H. Mayer | M. Nickl | C. Nickl-Weller | E. Oborn
N. Pilosof | H. Praetorius | S. Redecke | A.-K. Salich | T. Sahlmann
U. Schrader | E. Schultz | C. Wagenaar | T. Willemeit

 Medizinisch Wissenschaftliche Verlagsgesellschaft

The Editors

Prof. Christine Nickl-Weller
Nickl & Partner Architekten AG
Lindberghstraße 19
80939 München

Dipl.-Ing. Stefanie Matthys
European Network Architecture
for Health gGmbH
Wikingerufer 7
10555 Berlin

Dipl.-Ing. Tanja Eichenauer
European Network Architecture
for Health gGmbH
Wikingerufer 7
10555 Berlin

Prof. Dr. Cor Wagenaar
Expertise Center Architecture,
Urbanism and Health
University of Groningen
Eelkemastraat 40
9723ZW Groningen
The Netherlands

MWV Medizinisch Wissenschaftliche Verlagsgesellschaft mbH & Co. KG
Unterbaumstraße 4
10117 Berlin
www.mwv-berlin.de

ISBN 978-3-95466-805-2
ISSN 2976-1883

Bibliographic Information of the German National Library
The German National Library (Deutsche Nationalbibliothek) has listed this publication in its German National Bibliography. Detailed bibliographic information is available online at http://dnb.d-nb.de.

© MWV Medizinisch Wissenschaftliche Verlagsgesellschaft Berlin, 2024

This piece of work, including all of its individual parts, is protected under copyright. The rights established thereby, in particular those regarding translation, reprinting, oral presentations, extraction of illustrations and tables, broadcasting, microfilming or any other types of duplication or storage in data processing plants, remain reserved, even only for partial use.

The reproduction of common names, trade names, product names, etc., in this work, even without special permission, does not justify the assumption that such names should, in the sense of trademark and brand protection legislation, be regarded as free and therefore usable by anyone. In this publication, only the masculine form has generally been used for the generic naming of persons of any sex, unless stated otherwise. If a contributor wished to have specific gender formulations used in his/her respective text, we were more than happy to adopt them in his/her contribution.

The authors have attempted to make sure that the technical and subject-specific content was up-to-date at the time of going to press. Nevertheless, errors or misprints cannot entirely be ruled out. Especially in the case of medical articles, the publisher cannot accept any liability for recommendations on diagnostic or therapeutic procedures, instructions regarding certain dosages, types of application or treatment, and so on. Such information must be verified by the reader for their accuracy in each specific case in accordance with the information provided by the respective manufacturer's instructions and those found in other relevant literature. Errata, should any exist, can be downloaded at any time from the publisher's website.

Product/Project Management: Anja Faulenbach, Berlin
Translation support: Bridie France
Layout & typesetting: zweiband.media, Agentur für Mediengestaltung und -produktion GmbH, Berlin
Printing: ADverts printing house

Please address all comments and criticism to:
MWV Medizinisch Wissenschaftliche Verlagsgesellschaft mbH & Co. KG, Unterbaumstraße 4, 10117 Berlin, lektorat@mwv-berlin.de

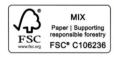

Introduction

"Efficient, modular and flexible structures" are key terms when it comes to formulating future challenges to building in the health care sector.

Health care and health infrastructure should be able to react quickly to changing needs. The pandemic has made this requirement even more pressing. The ideal of resource-efficient and patient-centred health care goes hand in hand with flexible adaptability. It is also an expression of increasingly digital and decentralised forms of care. To what extent can sustainability and architectural quality be brought into the design of quickly set up, modular and flexibly adaptable structures, and what is their place in the health care sector, which is generally focused on long-term developments? Can innovative construction methods and rethinking urban planning contribute to ensuring efficient, patient and lifestyle-oriented health care?

The 9th Symposium "Health Care of the Future" is dedicated to these questions by highlighting programmatic, social and structural aspects of future-oriented health care. It breaks the topic down into four thematic sessions:

- Flexible frameworks—Future-proof frameworks for adaptive health care systems
- Adaptive structures—Design solutions for innovative and flexible health care architecture
- Fix—recover—prevent—Contemporary concepts for a connected health landscape
- Responses to global crises—Design solutions to address pandemics and scarcity of resources

In addition to innovative best-practice examples from renowned architects, we will hear the opinions of thought leaders and scientists in the health care sector.

We look forward to stimulating contributions and good ideas for the health care of the future!

The Scientific Advisory Board of the European Network Architecture for Health
Reinhard Busse
Christine Nickl-Weller
Magnus Nickl
Lars Steffensen
Cor Wagenaar

Welcome

Almost two years ago, we met at the Academy of Arts in Berlin for the 9th Symposium Health Care of the Future entitled "Fast & Flexible—Planning adaptive structures in health care". We discussed the need to build a radical new health care system with radically redesigned hospitals. We had experienced two years of lockdown, and the coronavirus crisis was behind us at last. However, the joy of returning to normality was dampened by the shocking news about the beginning of the war in Ukraine—events that were unimaginable for me personally until then.

The title "Fast & Flexible" responded to the challenges and realisations of those last few years. The crises we had endured and were still facing made it clear how much the health care system needs to be able to react to the unforeseen. The coronavirus crisis brought health to the forefront of daily social and political interest, and every news report began with information on the current status of the pandemic and how to deal with it.

Never before has our health care system been so much in the public eye, while at the same time we realised that many of our hospitals were not up to these challenges. There was an obvious lack of further development and implementation of a digitally networked system; I am thinking here of a wide variety of platforms, some of which still do not co-operate to this day.

It has also become clear that the structural and technical conditions of our health care facilities are not conducive to reacting quickly in a crisis. There are many reasons for this, but they can often be found in building structures that allow little or no flexibility. At best, in recent decades, hospitals have been extended and newly built to fit perfectly within long-established structures. This rigid corset of hospital planning begins with the space allocation plan—tailor-made from past experience (from the 1970s). This is certainly due to a piecemeal approach to hospital planning rather than long-term systematic planning, as well as a lack of courage to make fundamental structural decisions about demand, networking and much more.

The contributions in this book, which are based on the presentations at the 9th symposium, are intended to create visions that give space to modularity and the interdisciplinarity that develops from it. These visions must question familiar, entrenched ways of doing things and deal openly with the question "Why not do it differently?".

By planning adaptive structures, we mean a reduction to three categories, for example: high-end diagnostics with therapy, high-end care and low care.

New ideas and concepts that could potentially expand the repertoire of current health care facilities are discussed in the articles that follow. Which forms of care could ensure better interconnection of the triad—healing, recovery, and prevention—in the future?

In the last part of the book, we take another look at the future. How can medicine and architecture work better, hand in hand, in the future, in order to be able to react quickly to global crisis situations? How can architecture be rethought in the future, possibly also against the backdrop of digitalised construction, in order to make better use of resources, both human and material? After all, the sustainable and environmentally friendly use of resources is essential for future developments in the construction sector.

Above all, however, we must not forget that the core of the intelligent health care system—the intelligent hospital—is humanity, despite all these challenges and endeavours towards networking and technological progress.

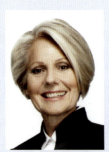

Prof. Christine Nickl-Weller

Nickl & Partner Architekten AG
München

ENAH
Berlin

Christine Nickl-Weller has been designing and realizing buildings for health, research and teaching as well as development and master plans since 1989. Since 2008 she was CEO of Nickl & Partner Architekten AG with offices in Munich, Berlin, Zurich, Beijing and Jakarta. In 2019 she became chairwoman of the board. As one of the leading offices in Germany in the field of medical facilities, clinics and research institutes, Nickl & Partner Architekten AG can refer to numerous national and international projects and awards.

From 2004 to 2018 Christine Nickl-Weller held the chair "Entwerfen von Krankenhäusern und Bauten des Gesundheitswesens" (now: Architecture for Health) at the Berlin University of Technology.

She initiated the symposium series "Health Care of the Future", which takes place biannually in Berlin. She is the editor and author of numerous books and articles, e.g. Healing Architecture (2013), Hospital Architecture (2013), Architecture for Health (2020), and the series Health Care of the Future 1-8 at Medizinisch Wissenschaftliche Verlagsgesellschaft.

Welcome

The 9th symposium "Health Care of the Future" once again addresses the big questions, and provides answers. Architects advertise with their achievements, and so it follows that the best-practice examples shown in the symposium provide a convincing stimulus and role model for the changing requirements of the health care sector.

"People shape spaces—spaces shape people"—nowhere else is this interaction felt as directly as in the health care sector. In hospitals, patients often have no choice but to spend days or weeks in the same room or to recuperate for a while in the outdoor facilities. It is therefore all the more important to create indoor and outdoor spaces for hospitals that respond to all the senses and promote the healing process. Likewise, the rooms must also serve doctors, nurses and other staff, both functionally and aesthetically. After all, physical and mental well-being is of paramount importance not only for patients, but also for all health care workers. We must ensure that inhospitable spaces do not encourage overwork and exhaustion. Open spaces and gardens are of particular importance here, especially during longer hospital stays.

The pandemic was not the first example of the need to meet a wide variety of requirements in order to be able to respond to current disease situations and their treatment methods. Modules and flexible construction methods, as well as outdoor spaces that can be adapted to different usage requirements, are central to doing so. And all of this, of course, should be done in a sustainable manner that is in harmony with our resources.

This great responsibility of architects of all disciplines in the health care sector must also be reflected in appropriate professional framework conditions, which the Federal Chamber of German Architects has been advocating since 1969. Fee scales, procurement regulations, sustainability requirements, digitalisation—the variety of topics is large and necessary in order to continue to be able to design spaces so that the people in them feel not only well, but better, and so that these spaces contribute to recovery.

My express thanks therefore go to all the organisers and participants of the 9th Symposium "Health Care of the Future", which has once again shown us what is possible in order to give people strength in their weakest moments.

Andrea Gebhard

Bundesarchitektenkammer (BAK)
Berlin

Andrea Gebhard was elected President of the Bundesarchitektenkammer (German Federal Chamber of Architects) on 28th May 2021. As a landscape architect and urban planner, Gebhard has been involved in professional politics for many years. In 1989, she became a member of the Bayerische Architektenkammer (Bavarian Chamber of Architects) and has been a member of the Bund Deutscher Landschaftsarchitekten (BDLA, Association of German Landscape Architects) since 1990. She was president of the BDLA from 2007 to 2013. Since 1999, she has been a member of the Deutsche Akademie für Städtebau und Landesplanung (DASL, German Academy for Urban and Regional Planning). She has also been a member of the Kuratorium für Nationale Stadtentwicklung (Board of Trustees for National Urban Development) since 2012. Since 2009, she has been co-owner of the office mahl gebhard konzepte.

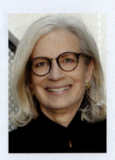

Welcome

On behalf of the TU Berlin, I would like to welcome you to the 9th Symposium "Health Care of the Future."

Some may wonder why the TU Berlin is sending its Vice President for Teacher Education and Young Academics to such an event. I have to admit: when I accepted the invitation for this welcome address last year, I was still hoping to also become Vice President for Sustainability and Transdisciplinarity at the TU from April onwards.

In the meantime, the TU has chosen a new beginning in leadership—and as of 1st April, Geraldine Rauch will lead a completely transformed TU Presidium as its new president. As head of the Institute for Biometry and Clinical Epidemiology and Vice Dean for Teaching at the Charité, Ms. Rauch is particularly close to the topics to be discussed today. I am therefore sure that you will continue to find contacts in the TU leadership who will emphatically support the European Network Architecture for Health.

When I first considered your invitation, I was, to be honest, not at all aware of the ground-breaking work in the Department of Architecture for Health at the TU Berlin—the work of Christine Nickl-Weller, of Lars Steffensen and their colleagues. However, I immediately found the vision you chose for this symposium series, which has been taking place since 2006, to be inspiring:

> *The symposium "Health Care of the Future" is based on the conviction that good architecture and urban planning can contribute to improve health care provision as well as prevention and health promotion.*

Unfortunately, as a patient, family member and visitor, I have often experienced the opposite of what is described in this positive vision: health care buildings that for me—even if one should not argue about taste—are often among the ugliest buildings in a city, and spaces that trigger an escape instinct rather than an increase in well-being.

How refreshing it is to deal with the ideas of a network whose goal is an architecture that places itself at the service of patients and healing. And at the same time (and as an economist I have a lot of sympathy for this) it also takes into account the requirements of efficiency and flexibility.

As a great believer in transdisciplinarity, I am delighted to see how this research paradigm is being brought to life in your network. Here, architects, urban planners, economists, physicians and other life scientists work together in an interdisciplinary way and with central actors from the practice of health care in order to jointly overcome complex societal challenges. In addition, the network lives up to its claim of being a European network, as the broad international background of the speakers and participants impressively demonstrates.

The great potential for the TU Berlin in such a collaboration becomes apparent when one realises that the largest increase in funding awarded by the German Research Foundation in recent years has been in the field of life sciences. Unfortunately, it is precisely in this area that the TU—as a university without a medical faculty or biology department—has so far had relatively little to offer. This makes it all the more important for established areas of the TU, such as architecture or economics, to collaborate with the life sciences at other research institutions. Our colleague Reinhard Busse is, after all, an important player in your network as head of the Department of Healthcare Management.

Looking at today's topics, I see a lot of further potential for cooperation with areas in which the TU is strong. For example, if we take the interconnected health care landscapes mentioned in Session 3 seriously, digitalisation plays a central role. Here, for example, we can think about increasing digital linkages between hospitals and patient care at home. The Corona pandemic has brought the potential of digitalisation to the attention of many people. Perhaps in the future, not only will gainful employment increasingly take place in the home office, but recovery will also take place more frequently in modern home health care. There should be exciting research opportunities on topics related to digitalisation, for example with colleagues from the Einstein Center Digital Future or the Weizenbaum Institute for the Networked Society, in which the TU is involved.

Regardless of whether health care takes place at home or in a hospital, questions of the psychological well-being of patients will hopefully play an increasing role in the future, also and especially within a highly technical health care system. Here I see the potential for collaboration between architecture for health and medical technology as well as psychology that deals with human-machine interactions—these are also areas in which the TU Berlin is strongly positioned.

As a university lecturer in economic education and sustainable consumption, I personally find it particularly positive and remarkable that your network not only strives for a balance between economic and social requirements, but that ecological issues are also taken centrally into consideration. With this multidimensionality, you create the prerequisite for finding truly viable, sustainable solutions, which is what today is all about. I am pleased that the TU Berlin now has a great deal to offer in the field of sustainable construction, sustainable infrastructure and energy supply, as well as sustainable materials and the circular economy in numerous specialist areas, so that there is also further potential for cooperation here.

With this in mind, I am very pleased that your conference is taking place in cooperation with the TU Berlin and I wish you many inspiring presentations and discussions. All the best in making the inspiring vision of your network a reality!

Prof. Dr. Ulf Schrader

Technische Universität Berlin

Ulf Schrader was Vice President for Teacher Education and Junior Scholars at Technische Universität Berlin from 2021 to 2022. He has been Professor of Economic Education and Sustainable Consumption at TU Berlin since 2008. From 2016 to 2021, he was also the Director of the School of Education of TU Berlin (SETUB). His main teaching and research focus has been on sustainable consumption, consumer education, and corporate social responsibility. He is a member of the Editorial Boards of the *Journal of Consumer Policy* and the *Journal Sustainability: Science, Practice and Policy*. Schrader has also been a member of the Scientific Advisory Board of the Bundesministerium für Ernährung, Landwirtschaft und Verbraucherschutz (German Federal Ministry for Nutrition, Agriculture and Consumer Protection), and a member of the Innovation Advisory Board of the Bundesministerium für wirtschaftliche Zusammenarbeit (German Federal Ministry for Economic Cooperation and Development).

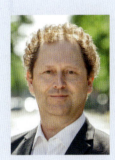

Contents

I Flexible Frameworks — 1

    Introduction — 3
    Thomas Willemeit

    1 Digital Technologies — A Key Driver for the Transformation of German Health Care — 5
       Jörg F. Debatin

    2 Methodical Procedure for Regional Structural Changes in the Hospital Sector — Examples from Denmark — 11
       Carolina Lohfert Praetorius and Henrik Praetorius

    3 Hôpital Universitaire Saint-Ouen Grand Paris Nord — 19
       Jérôme Brunet and Thorsten Sahlmann

II Adaptive Structures — 33

    Introduction — 35

    1 Future Cities Health Care Ecosystems — Digitally Enabling Hybrid Care Models across Physical and Virtual Environments — 37
       Nirit Pilosof, Eivor Oborn and Michael Barrett

    2 The Role of Building Services in the Resilient and Zero Carbon Future of Health Care Design — 47
       Frank Jensen

    3 The Hospital of the Future — 55
       Reinier de Graaf

III Fix — Recover — Prevent — 63

    Introduction — 65
    Sebastian Redecke

    1 Circle of Health — Expanding Berlin's Medical Care — 67
       Ann-Kathrin Salich

    2 Modular Solutions for a Sustainable Future — 75
       Magnus Nickl

Contents

IV Responses to global crises — 83

Introduction — 85
Cor Wagenaar

1 A Safe Environment to Look Micro and Design Macro — The WHO Technical Science for Health Network — 89
Michele Di Marco and Luca Fontana

2 Sustainable Futures — Digital Technologies — 95
Hannes Mayer

3 Structure and Synthesis — 103
Edzard Schultz

Closing Words — 111
Stefanie Matthys

Science in Dialogue with Industry — 113

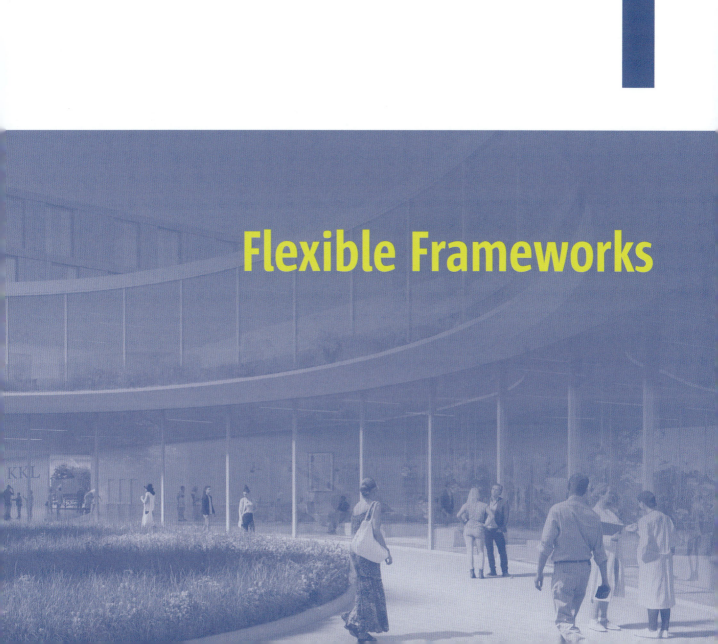

Flexible Frameworks

I

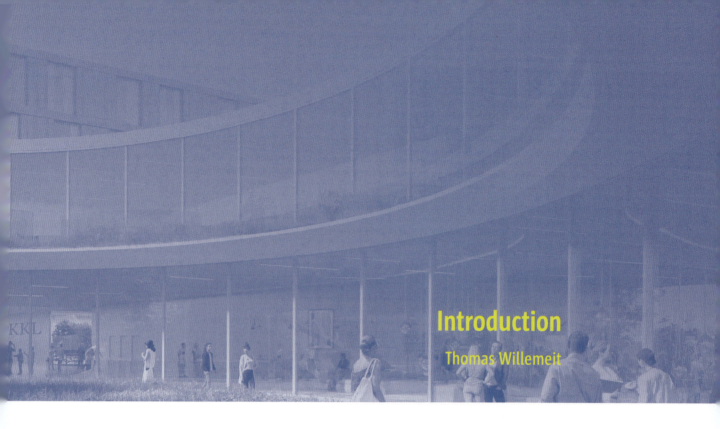

Introduction

Thomas Willemeit

Over the past couple of years, during the Corona crisis, health care has moved to the centre of our attention. In particular, digitalisation has benefited from new developments, and the acceptance of apps and remote observation has grown. More and more, we are talking about "home medicine" and "home hospital", remote control and treatment. The fact that fifty or sixty participants are now joining us from their offices remotely is emblematic of that shift. But this is just the tip of the iceberg, a symptom of disruptive societal change and a driver of the transformation of our healing environments.

The big trailblazer Eric Topol speculated on digitalisation in medicine in his famous book *The Patient Will See You Now*. The title of his publication predicts that patients should and will become the masters of their data in the cloud. Due to the fact that diagnostics can take place online as well, information is now much more transparent and accessible for patients. This pushes people to centre stage. Digitalisation provides us with ever more precise imaging processes, analytics, diagnostics, and internationally comparative medicine. So, physicians supported by AI are in a different place now as well. New technologies and rituals require different spaces and at the end of the day, health care architecture will also be dramatically influenced by digitalisation.

Mr. Topol argues that doctors will ultimately be able to spend more time with their patients because diagnostics is supported by AI and is therefore becoming faster. We hope that things will move this way. We are the precursors and the trailblazers in the way we devise architecture.

Many of our colleagues—architects—have already dealt with the impact of digitalisation on work and retail environments. Traditional typologies in architecture are in a process of transformation, influenced by digital communication, administration and commerce. Now this will also increasingly play a very important role in health care. There is going to be a disruptive change spurred by digitalisation.

I Flexible Frameworks

How aggressively will we concentrate on health care competences? Do we need decentralised, small health hubs? Will outpatient centres be bigger? What about telemedicine? Will it take over completely? This takes me to the topic of the first session, with the title "Flexible frameworks." We have got a fantastic international panel and we will learn how health care environments are currently designed in Denmark, in Germany, and in France.

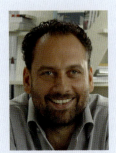

Dipl.-Ing. Arch. Thomas Willemeit

GRAFT Gesellschaft von Architekten mbH
Berlin

Thomas Willemeit studied architecture at the Technische Universität Braunschweig, where he graduated as Dipl.-Ing. Arch. in 1997, and took part in the masterclass for architecture and urban planning at the Bauhaus Dessau. Alongside his successful career in the architectural field, he has won numerous national prizes as a violin player and a chorister. He was Visiting Professor for Architecture at the RWTH Aachen and at Peter Behrens School of Art in Düsseldorf and has also been a visiting professor at the Technische Universität Delft in 2017–18. In 1998, Thomas Willemeit established GRAFT in Los Angeles, together with Lars Krückeberg and Wolfram Putz. With further offices in Berlin and Shanghai, GRAFT has been commissioned to design and manage a wide range of projects. Since its foundation, GRAFT has won numerous national and international awards and has earned an international reputation. Thomas Willemeit, Lars Krückeberg and Wolfram Putz, together with Marianne Birthler, curated the German Pavilion in Venice at the Architecture Biennale 2018.

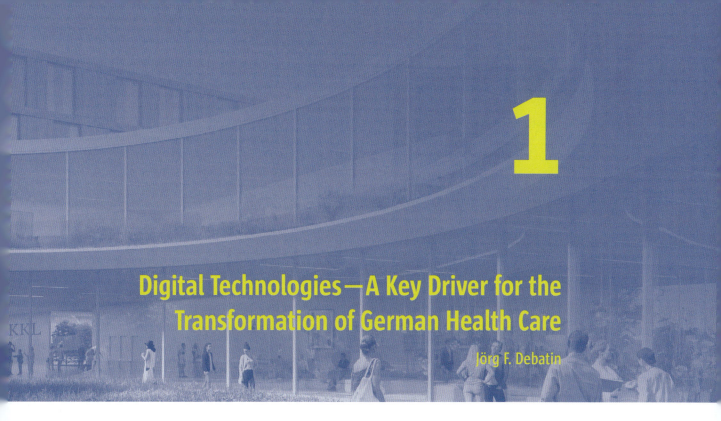

1

Digital Technologies—A Key Driver for the Transformation of German Health Care

Jörg F. Debatin

The implementation and use of digital technologies in medicine aim at improving outcome quality and efficiency, thereby creating value for patients and health care providers alike. These benefits became evident during the Corona pandemic. Thanks to video consultations, patients could virtually bring their doctor right into their living room. This led to more safety (as they did not have to expose themselves to the viruses of other patients in the waiting room), more comfort, and more efficiency.

Digital technologies can be important building blocks to improve the quality and productivity of healthcare. In view of the ongoing demographic change, health care must become more efficient. Digital technologies are also needed to harvest the benefits based on the decoding of human biology. Thus, personalised medicine on a molecular basis requires the handling of millions of differentiation criteria per cell. To identify the optimal therapy for each individual, appropriate digital tools must be employed.

Interestingly, the population in general has high expectations regarding the utility of digital tools in a healthcare environment. An overwhelming majority agrees on the benefits of digital medicine. This acceptance of digital technologies among the population was also the incentive for a veritable firework-display of legal activities in the last legislative period in Germany, with Jens Spahn as Minister of Health. Central—and long overdue—legal foundations were created. A total of twenty-eight laws were passed, six of which focused on digital medical content; the Social Code had to be amended forty-five times. Thanks to these diverse initiatives, it was possible to make up a little for what had been left unaddressed in Germany in the previous fifteen years.

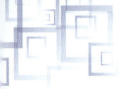

| Flexible Frameworks

Foundations for the Digital Transformation

What has been done? The first step was to create a foundation for the implementation of digital technologies. The central basis for any use of digital data is its interoperability. What good is more data if it doesn't communicate with each other? Unfortunately, Germany has so far been characterised primarily by the use of proprietary, i.e., company-specific, data formats. Recent legislative efforts have addressed the deficit: the use of international standards has now become mandatory in Germany for digital medical data. These include FHIR standards for data formats and SNOMED CT for semantics.

The next step is to create a basis for connectivity. This was created with the so-called telematics infrastructure (TI). All healthcare providers were connected via a specially protected data highway. This reflects the special nature of medical data, which does require special protection. The telematics infrastructure has now connected all 180,000 physicians in private practice, all hospitals, as well as all pharmacies. It is being rolled out to other health care providers including therapists, care institutions and ambulatory nursing organisations. The digitalisation agency Gematik, in which the federal government now holds a majority stake, is overseeing this process.

Interoperability and connectivity have laid the groundwork for digital applications. The first application regulates the secure digital exchange of patient-related data between service providers, for example, between a specialist and a general practitioner or between a hospital and a general practitioner. With KIM (Communication in Medicine), the time-honoured fax was replaced. With KIM, the German health care system has a secure e-mail structure. TIM, a secure messaging system, is to follow in 2023. The initial focus will be on communication between pharmacists and physicians, between specialists and general practitioners, and many others.

A second application is the electronic reporting of periods of incapacity for work and previous illness. About seventy-seven million of these certificates are issued in Germany every year, and when you consider that each one costs fifteen minutes of time, it's perfectly clear that digitalisation offers huge potential savings. The new system is already connected and in use. From January 2023, the use of this digital application will be mandatory.

Digital Apps become Part of Standard Care

Until now, doctors have been able to prescribe medicines and remedies, for example, crutches and the like. These have now been joined by apps, or DiGAs (digital health apps), which help patients to advance their health—for example, in the convalescence process—by using digital tools on their smart-phones. Taking the example of a hip replacement: the patient receives a prescription for physiotherapy once or twice a week. With the help of an app, guided exercises can be performed and documented multiple times each day. The app measures, gives individualised instructions, and much more.

This concept was developed in 2019. Within one legislative session, the idea was successfully translated from conceptualisation and parliamentary approval to clinical reality. In the meantime, more than thirty DiGAs have been listed as reimbursable by the Federal Institute for Drugs and Medical Devices (BfArM).

In Germany, there are two stages that medical devices must pass through before being placed on the market. First, the safety of the product must be proven. An Apple watch, for example, is not a medical device, because Apple has not yet wanted to undergo this testing. If the product is reliable, the BfArM checks whether it is beneficial. In the case of medical apps, this second analysis regarding the actual value could be based on a well-founded bene-

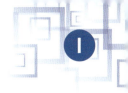

fit hypothesis. While this hypothesis must be backed up with data, it does not require final proof for the app to be put into circulation. A DiGA can initially be made available in this way for 12 months. The developers can use this time to gather the evidence necessary to prove their hypotheses and thereby permanently list the app.

DiGAs have now been prescribed 100,000 times. That's a small number, but given the fact that the first prescription only started in October 2020, the numbers do show that this innovation is making its way. It is encouraging that 60 percent of primary care physicians are positive about the program and want to prescribe DiGAs as well. It has been especially worthwhile for people with psychosocial problems, depression, tinnitus and much more.

"E-prescription" is coming soon. The current time-consuming, paper-based process is due to be replaced by digital prescription. From a medical point of view, e-prescription will bring enormous progress, as they will provide an overview of what medications have dispensed to an individual patient. The availability of such an overview will significantly strengthen drug therapy safety.

The foundation for much of what digital medicine has to offer is the electronic patient record. It should contain everything that is relevant to the patient's health. Both patients and doctors will be able to enter relevant information into this file. Here, too, there are considerable delays in implementation.

The new German government wants to help speed up its implementation. The main issue here is data privacy, as the new coalition government has promised in its coalition agreement that everyone will get an electronic patient record, except for those who object. This is what is referred to as "opt-out." Until now, the rule has been "opt-in", requiring patients to actively ask for an electronic patient record. In the future, it will work the other way around.

Digital Transformation of German Hospitals

Digitalisation in hospitals was also lagging in Germany. There are highly convincing studies that document how the implementation of digital tools can improve healthcare outcomes and at the same time generate huge savings in hospitals. The Universitätsklinikum Hamburg-Eppendorf showed how it could have been done many years ago. The hospital has been operating completely paper-free since 2010. Even twelve years after implementation, it still benefits medical outcomes and improves efficiency.

Unfortunately, there have been too few imitators. This became clear during the Corona pandemic when the number of available intensive care beds could not be readily answered. The fact that all data had to be recorded manually triggered the Hospital Future Act (KhZG). It was financed with 3 billion euros from the federal government, and with an additional 1.3 billion euros from the states.

The Hospital Future Act is a well-drafted law in which ten fields of digital transformation are clearly defined. The legislation focusses on "essentials", such as patient portals, bed planning, digital files, and secure medication supply. For each of these areas, there are mandatory criteria that must be met in order to receive funding. In addition, there are optional criteria.

The impact of the law on the digital maturity of German hospitals will be measured. An initial measurement among 1,600 hospitals revealed a digital maturity level of 33.7 points out of 100. As an initial finding, these poor results underscore the need to catch up. The measurement will be repeated in two years' time.

On the one hand, the KhZG has funding incentives, while on the other hand, hospitals that are still not sufficiently digitalised by 1st January 2025 will be subject to billing penalties. This form of legislation has led all hospitals to

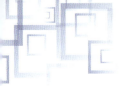

place the issue of digitalisation high on their agenda.

Reforming the German Hospital Landscape

The German hospital landscape is characterised by too many small hospitals with too many beds in total. In addition, recent years have shown a decline in the number of inpatients. Compared with 2019, there was a 15 percent decline in 2021. Together with the acute shortage of nurses and doctors, this is leading to acute financial difficulties in many hospitals.

The policy response is clear: concentrate services and close hospitals. At first glance, this sounds logical, but it becomes problematic in individual cases. One such individual case from my immediate environment is exemplified by two hospitals in the north of Essen, which were closed because it is well documented that there are sufficient hospitals in the south of Essen.

This is true, and what's more, the hospitals in the south are also of better quality. Nevertheless, there were protests, because people wanted local care. With the closures, many citizens felt left behind. The result: in the local elections, there was a considerable strengthening of the extreme fringes within our party spectrum. So, we have a political dilemma. Logical decisions regarding hospital infrastructure do not reflect the wishes of the population.

On the subject of quality, it should be noted that quality does not always have to be centralised. This logic comes into play in cardiac surgery. Competence and skills must be available centrally in one place, since physical presence is required. However, there are also many cases where virtually available competencies and skills are sufficient. This applies, for example, to radiology, laboratory services, consulting and much more.

A prerequisite for a decentralised solution is the availability of digital technology on-site. To import "off-site" high quality medical know-how and experience, digital applications, data transfer, as well as digital communication and documentation must be available. Worth mentioning here is the Technical University in Munich, which is not only pioneering in the field of architecture, but also in the field of technology. Here they are working on miniaturisation of measuring devices, so-called "POC – Point of Care" and "Home Health", i.e., in areas where convalescence at home works better than in the hospital.

Tele-Medicine Can Even Support Intensive Care

An example, which also worked during the pandemic, was tele-ICU. Experts not only used their knowledge for the benefit of the intensive care patients in their hospitals, but also provided care for smaller hospitals. They went on rounds with mobile robots. Issues relating to liability and data protection were quickly raised, which in turn were quickly resolved, thanks to Corona.

The company TCC (Telehealth Competence Center) in Hamburg has taken this approach even further. They have set up command centres in which they provide telemedical care for intensive care patients in various hospitals and intensive care units. Results from three hospitals working with TCC show that clinical care is not only improving, but that ICU stays are also being reduced.

Back to the north of Essen. Citizens want to be cared for in an emergency and wish to be taken care of with minor illnesses. For serious injuries, as well as heart attacks and strokes, Germany relies on sophisticated rescue chains. It is mostly about the minor emergencies. It's about the sprained foot that you don't know whether it's broken or not. In such a case, people want on-site outpatient care, 24/7. A "simple" illness can then be cared for on-site. If it is a serious diagnosis, people are willing to seek specialised therapy is at an institution that is farther away.

For these medical purposes I advocate the "DigiMax" clinic concept for on-site care. Emergency assessment for minor injuries is provided with 24/7 availability. Diagnostic services are offered that are maximally equipped in terms of technology. While collected locally, the data are analysed off-site. The same can be accomplished for laboratory and other forms of monitoring. Physical exams need to involve more established structures. Nursing stations are needed, for patients where the focus is less on medical procedures and more on nursing care, and should be available for stays up to forty-eight hours. People expect these medical services to be available close by. Instead of closing hospitals, we should consider their transformation to "DigiMax" clinics, that provide high quality medicine based on tele-technologies.

The Future

The digital transformation of the healthcare system in Germany has begun. Foundations have been laid. Several major applications such as e-prescriptions and the implementation of a workable electronic patient record must follow. This also applies to hospitals, which have a lot of work ahead of them in the next two years. Hospital planning should focus more on people's needs. As I mentioned, digitalisation is not an end in itself, but neither is hospital planning. We all serve patients and their needs. All those who ignore this, as we have seen very vividly in the example of Essen, will suffer political consequences. We need alternatives to closure, such as the transformation to DigiMax clinics.

The incredible suffering in Ukraine dwarfs all our problems including our challenges in the health sector. In this regard, it is worth highlighting that there is a special relationship with Ukraine regarding the digital transformation of the health sector, as many digital architects and digital implementers come from Ukraine. Many innovations would not be possible without these digital experts.

| This text was transliterated by Tanja Eichenauer.

Prof. Dr. med. Jörg F. Debatin, MBA

Healthcare-Entrepreneur
Mülheim an der Ruhr

Until December 2021 Jörg F. Debatin was Chairman of the Health Innovation Hub of the Federal Ministry of Health, Berlin. Prior to that he served as Vice President and CTO for GE Healthcare in Waukesha, USA (2014–2018), and CEO of amedes Holding AG in Germany (2011–2014). From 2003–2011 he led the University Medical Center Hamburg-Eppendorf as its Medical Director and CEO. Having been trained as a diagnostic Radiologist at Duke and Staford, he was appointed full Professor of Diagnostic Radiology at the University Medical Center of Essen in 1998.

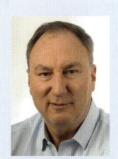

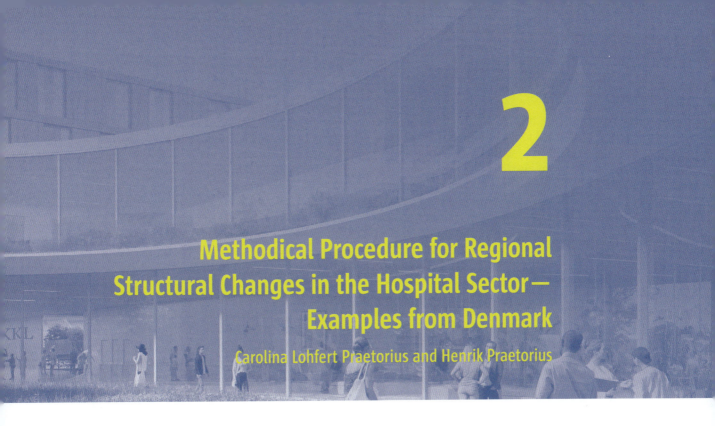

Methodical Procedure for Regional Structural Changes in the Hospital Sector — Examples from Denmark

Carolina Lohfert Praetorius and Henrik Praetorius

Structural changes in the hospital sector

Structural changes in the hospital system will be an important and essential topic in Germany in the coming years. A comparison of the health care systems in Denmark and Germany shows differences with regard to the interface between outpatient and inpatient care. In Germany, these areas are more separate than in Denmark.

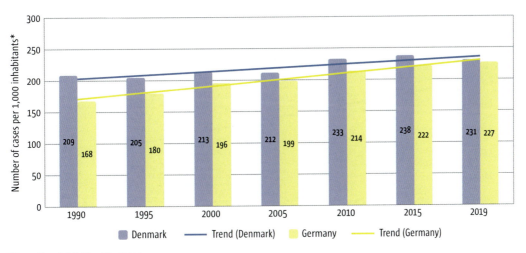

*General hospitals (without Psychiatry)

Fig. 1 Number of cases per 1,000 inhabitants (Denmark: Sundhedsstyrelsen, Sygehusstatik. Sundhedsdata, Statens Serum Institut; Germany: Statistisches Bundesamt [http://www.destatis.de], Grunddaten der Krankenhäuser)

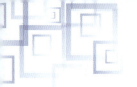

| Flexible Frameworks

In Denmark, the 2007 health care reform led to major structural changes in the health care system as well as modernisation of hospital buildings. Care regions were merged and the number of hospitals reduced, resulting in greater centralisation of specialist care. The aim of the structural changes was to establish forward-looking and flexible hospitals with a focus on quality. In addition, the length of patients' stay in hospital was to be further reduced and services were to be shifted to outpatient departments. Overall, follow-up cost savings of 8% were expected after the new buildings were put into operation.

Comparison of the health care systems Denmark and Germany

People's average life span is approximately the same in Germany and Denmark; patients are basically equally ill and are treated to the same extent (s. fig. 1).

Health care spending in Germany and Denmark as a share of gross domestic product (GDP) has risen in recent years, primarily due to the COVID-19 pandemic. In Germany, spending is around 1% higher than in Denmark. In Denmark, about 85% of health care spending is recovered through taxes and 15% through private co-payments. In Germany, there are statutory health insurance funds and state co-payments, which also finance 85% of costs.

However, the hospital structure is very different. There are almost three times as many beds per inhabitant in Germany than in Denmark: 2.0 beds in Denmark vs. 5.4 beds in Germany per 1,000 inhabitants in 2019, excluding psychiatry (s. fig. 2). The average length of stay in hospital (excluding psychiatry) is more than twice as high in Germany at 6.6 days compared to Denmark, where the length of stay is 2.9 days (s. fig. 3). Since 2010, there have been about three times as many hospitals per million inhabitants in Germany as in Denmark (s. fig. 4).

Methodical procedure for regional structural changes

The 2007 health care reform in Denmark reduced hospital planning units from 14 to 5 by combin-

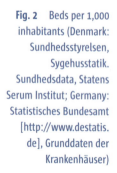

Fig. 2 Beds per 1,000 inhabitants (Denmark: Sundhedsstyrelsen, Sygehusstatik. Sundhedsdata, Statens Serum Institut; Germany: Statistisches Bundesamt [http://www.destatis.de], Grunddaten der Krankenhäuser)

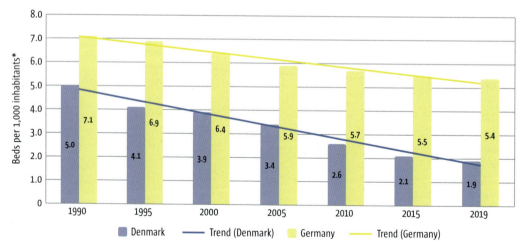

*General hospitals (without Psychiatry)

2 Methodical Procedure for Regional Structural Changes in the Hospital Sector—Examples from Denmark

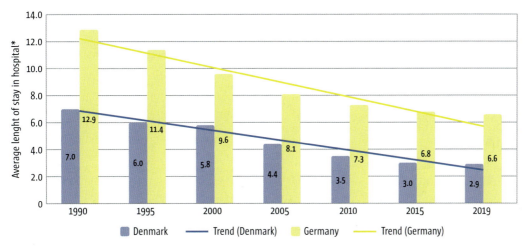

Fig. 3 Average length of stay in hospital (Denmark: Sundhedsstyrelsen, Sygehusstatik. Sundhedsdata, Statens Serum Institut; Germany: Statistisches Bundesamt [http://www.destatis.de], Grunddaten der Krankenhäuser)

*General hospitals (without Psychiatry)

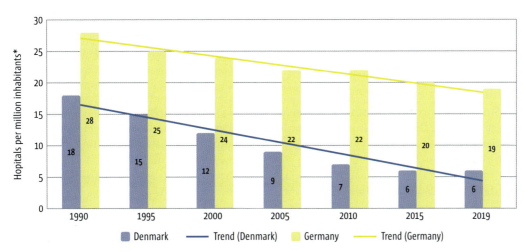

Fig. 4 Hospitals per million inhabitants

*General hospitals (without Psychiatry)

ing larger service regions (s. fig. 5). The number of acute care hospitals was to be reduced from 64 to 22, and at the same time large investments were to be made in hospital buildings in order to complete new buildings or carry out conversions.

The following guiding principles underpinned the structural changes to Denmark's hospital system:
- Quality takes precedence over proximity
- Better utilisation of economic and professional resources
- Planning of interdisciplinary emergency rooms (basis 200,000–400,000 inhabitants)

| Flexible Frameworks

Fig. 5 Change in Hospital Structure 2007–2022

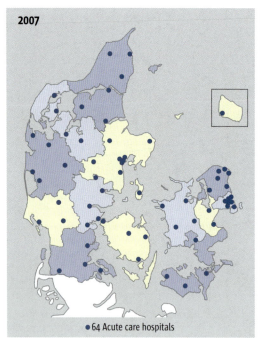
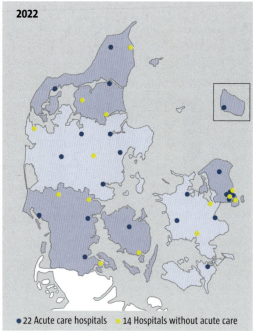

- Shifting services to the outpatient sector (50%), which should result in a 20% reduction in beds

Each service region had the task of developing master plans incorporating the guiding principles. Building-functional analyses of the sites, performance and capacity calculations, and medical enterprise plans were developed. Building master plans summarised building options for medical structural changes.

The individual hospital projects in each region were assessed by a panel of experts from a Quality Fund set up by the government. The expert jury was asked to prepare opinions and assess the extent to which the goals would be implemented in the regions. For example, the expert jury assessed whether the merging of hospitals was in accordance with medical quality standards. New construction and remodelling plans should also be effective and economical.

The length of patients' stay in hospital was to be further reduced and services were to be shifted to hospitals' outpatient departments. Overall, follow-up cost savings of 8% were expected after the new buildings were put into operation. The investment for the projects was only approved if these targets could be achieved.

The restructuring of the hospitals was mainly implemented through new buildings or large extensions, so that space usage standards were implemented in a future-oriented manner. In Denmark, there were still hospitals that had five-bed and six-bed rooms without a bathroom. As part of the health care reform, it was decided that only one-bed rooms with their own bathroom should be built in order to increase patient safety and thus reduce the number of infections acquired in hospital. A further priority was confidentiality in conversations between patients and staff.

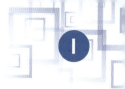

2 Methodical Procedure for Regional Structural Changes in the Hospital Sector—Examples from Denmark

The goal was to create a hospital system with modern, flexible, effective and economical hospitals with a focus on quality. Optimal conditions were to be created with regard to the following:
- Better organisation of coherent patient workflows
- Optimisation of workflows through the use of new technology and innovations in the health care sector
- Reduced transport of patients, staff, and goods between hospitals
- Rationalisation of on-call services, laboratory functions, X-ray, etc.
- Better utilisation of radiological equipment, etc.
- Centralisation of administrative and technical functions

As part of the reform, the government launched an investment program in 2007 to modernise hospitals and provided funds totalling around 5.5 billion euros (price basis 2007). Some of the new buildings are now in operation, others will follow in the coming years.

Example: The capital region of Copenhagen

The capital region of Copenhagen, with a total population of around two million, was divided into four sub-regions, each of which was to provide care for 300,000–550,000 inhabitants. Seven hospitals were closed, and one acute care hospital was to be provided in each subregion. In the larger sub-regions, partner hospitals were established in which planned treatments were to be carried out. In total, approximately 4,200 beds were to be provided in the capital region of Copenhagen (s. fig. 6).

Each subregion should provide primary care for patients. Low-volume specialist care should be provided at only one hospital in the region or, in the case of higher volume, at two hospitals in the region.

A new building in Hillerød, in the north of the capital region of Copenhagen, has been planned on a greenfield site and will be in operation in 2025. At all other sites in the region, the plans were mostly extensions to existing sites. A large extension at Rigshospital was commissioned in 2020. A large paediatric clinic will be completed at Rigshospital in 2026. A new building at Herlev Hospital was commissioned in 2022. A new building at Glostrup Hospital will be completed in 2023, a new building at Hvidovre Hospital will be completed in 2024, and a new building at Bispebjerg Hospital will be completed in 2026.

What have we learned?

The investment backlog that existed in many hospitals was largely eliminated with the new construction projects. Old hospital structures often have a space deficit, e.g., insufficient ancillary areas. The new buildings have made it possible to improve space usage and to dismantle old pavilion structures. The optimisation of operational organisation which was made possible by new buildings, e.g., through standardised ward sizes, also allows flexibility in terms of construction.

The goal of the structural reform—to reduce the total number of beds by 20% through the centralisation of the hospital structure—has been surpassed with a total reduction of 25%. Outpatient visits were to be expanded by 50%, and that goal has long been achieved as well. There has been a very large shift of services from inpatient to outpatient care.

What was not adequately considered was the additional cost of organisational adjustments and relocation to the new hospitals.

It is essential to establish a highly digitalised wayfinding system. The system is very well de-

I Flexible Frameworks

Fig. 6 Changes in the capital region of Copenhagen

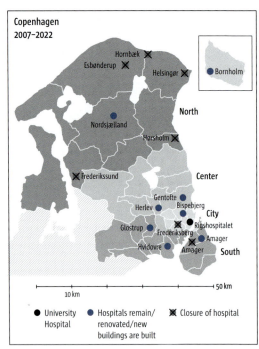 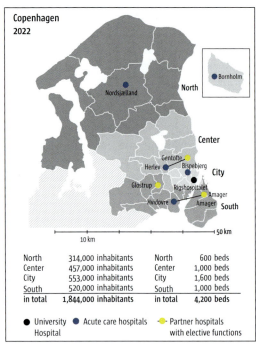

veloped in Denmark, so that patients are guided to the right hospital and waiting times for acute treatment are short. Surveys on patient satisfaction are carried out on an ongoing basis. In general, they show a very high level of satisfaction. Patients are prepared to travel further in order to receive better treatment.

We have learned that centralisation actually leads to an improvement in care. Although the catchment areas become larger, specialised hospitals and focus centres increase the number of specialist staff in the hospital. Patients are treated where the best expertise is. Since these "super hospitals" started operating in Denmark, the improved quality of treatment has led to higher patient satisfaction. More efficient treatment has significantly reduced patients' length of stay in hospital and increased the number of outpatient treatments.

Structural changes in the hospital system will be an important and essential topic in Germany in the coming years in order to achieve modern, flexible, effective and economical hospitals in which patients receive high quality treatment.

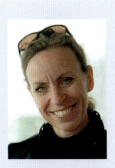

Carolina Lohfert Praetorius

Lohfert – Praetorius A/S
Kongens Lyngby
Denmark

Carolina Lohfert Praetorius is CEO of LOHFERT – PRAETORIUS A/S. She is a trained physician and has a Masters in Communication. Having worked as a project manager for more than 15 years, she has extensive experience from some 100 hospital projects in Denmark, Norway, Germany, Switzerland and Austria. Carolina Lohfert Praetorius has in-depth knowledge of all phases of hospital planning, especially in structural planning, capacity calculations, spatial planning, functional analysis, operational organisation planning, and commissioning planning as well as investment and follow-up cost calculations. Carolina Lohfert Praetorius is an expert in the planning, management and realisation of hospital planning projects.

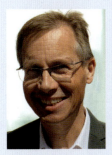

Henrik Praetorius

Lohfert – Praetorius A/S
Kongens Lyngby
Denmark

After more than 25 years with LOHFERT – PRAETORIUS A/S, Henrik Praetorius has a high level of expertise in and comprehensive knowledge of all aspects of hospital planning. During his time with LOHFERT – PRAETORIUS A/S, Henrik Praetorius has realised over 200 hospital planning projects in Denmark, Norway, Germany and Austria. Henrik Praetorius is an expert in the field of hospital planning and has extensive experience in project management as well as in all phases of hospital planning, most importantly functional analysis and planning, capacity calculation, spatial planning, and logistics planning as well as investment and follow-up cost calculations.

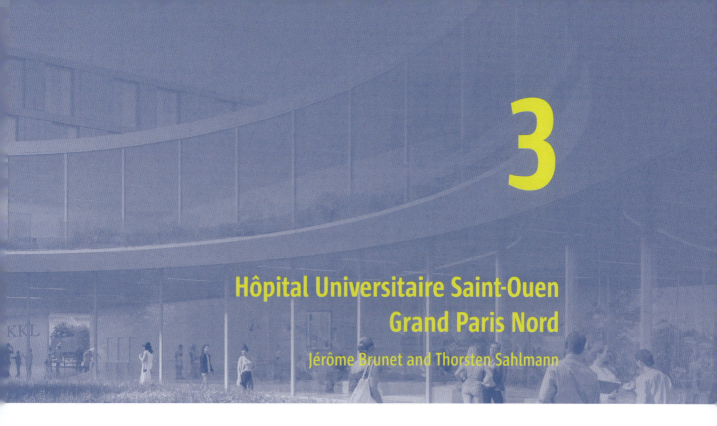

3

Hôpital Universitaire Saint-Ouen Grand Paris Nord

Jérôme Brunet and Thorsten Sahlmann

Care machine

Its code name mentions that it is located in Saint-Ouen, but constitutes a new infrastructure for the whole of Greater Paris North, hence its very large size: 160,000 m².

The notion of a "machine à soigner" ("care machine") refers to Le Corbusier's "machine à habiter" ("machine for living in"). This term, often misinterpreted, did not mean that he was building "machines" in which to live, but expressed the method of building these dwellings, inspired by the engineer of the time, who was developing transatlantic ships, aeroplanes and automobiles in large quantities. Today, we think of the hospital as a process. This does not mean that the hospital is a factory. Some may find that the rigorous concept of the structural framework on which we base our projects de facto inscribes them with an aesthetic and habitability that is more industrial than convivial. This is also a misinterpretation of the term "care machine" as simply a design method.

Figure 1 illustrates the typology of the Bichat hospital (top left). It is composed of a technical base on which residential blocks are placed. The Beaujon hospital (top right) is a vertical building. Built in the 1930s, at the same time as the Edouard Herriot hospital in Lyon designed by Tony Garnier on a pavilion plan that was classic for the time, this quasi-New York brick tower reverses the traditional horizontal model and proposes a superposition of floors, on each of which there is a part of the technical platform (an area with high technical infrastructure) and accommodation (hospital wards). One can imagine the contrast that this construction could produce at that time in the surrounding suburban fabric.

The Grand Paris-Nord University Hospital (HUSOGPN) in Saint-Ouen (below) shows the abandonment of the specificity of space by proposing a continuum in three dimensions within which the different functions are arranged. Their proximity, superimpositions and connections are evolving, in particular dur-

I Flexible Frameworks

Fig. 1 Archetype, scale, and grid

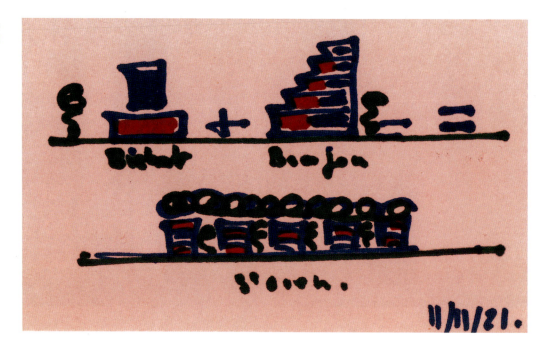

ing the early design phase with the client, the medical staff and the users. A hospital takes an average of twelve years from the first sketches to delivery. The programme evolves during the course of the project, as does medicine, which inevitably means that changes have to be incorporated throughout the design process to ensure that the building is not obsolete by the time it is completed. Hence the idea of creating a neutral, generic and unmarked space, in the positive sense of the word.

Then comes the notion of scale. Figure 2 shows the footprint of the future HUSOGPN placed on top of the Palais Royal in Paris. The very large size is one of the important assets of this project. Putting a garden of this size on the roof of a hospital offers a protected outdoor space, dedicated not only to the nursing staff and patients, but also to the neighbourhood and the inhabitants of Saint-Ouen and the surrounding area. This gesture is also a response to opening up to the city, to respond to the current paradox of wanting to be connected while, at the same time, access controls to public facilities are being reinforced.

The Bichat and Beaujon hospitals probably originally planned large green areas with trees around the buildings. Today, parking and service areas have replaced the lawns and trees. By placing the garden on the roof of the HUSOGPN, we prevent the colonisation of the green spaces, which are a source of well-being and spatial, environmental and social quality of the project, by a car park or an access road. It is no longer a "free" or vacant space, but an integral part of the hospital.

3 Hôpital Universitaire Saint-Ouen Grand Paris Nord

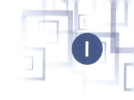

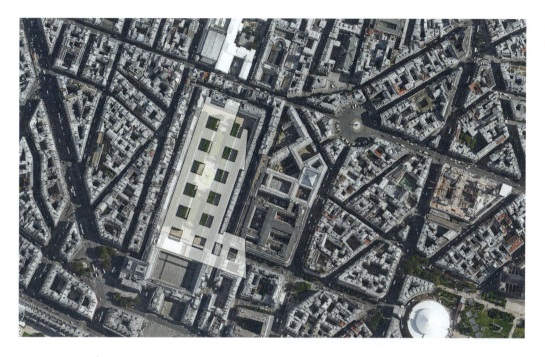

Fig. 2 Collage: footprint of the project on top of the Palais Royal

Neutral grid

Together with the architect Gerold Zimmerli, Brunet Saunier & Associés developed the continuum concept back in 2001, which, in contrast to previous hospitals, no longer distinguishes between specific functions such as the technical platform (area with a concentration of technical infrastructure), accommodation (wards), logistics or other services. The rapid development of medicine is changing the medical processes and the length of stay. The area dedicated to accommodation in the hospital is decreasing, to the benefit of the more and better equipped technical platform, consultation rooms and the day clinic. Our proposal is to no longer differentiate programmes by function, but to create a neutral infrastructure within which functions can be arranged, regardless of their nature.

Everything starts from a grid, which spreads over the area and meets the limits of the site (s. fig. 3 and 4).

We then place what we call the invariants (the points of ascent, the emergency staircases, the technical shafts) at the optimal regulatory distances to limit their number. This generic skeleton then constitutes the rigid framework of the project, the rule from which the functions can be freely deployed (s. fig. 5).

The floors are regularly pierced by generous patios to bring natural light into the heart of the building (s. fig. 6). The large size of these interior courtyards and the fact that they are planted filters the view while allowing one patio to be distinguished from another.

The central axis of each level groups the various vertical circulations. Accessed on both sides, this layout offers the possibility of a dou-

I Flexible Frameworks

Fig. 3   Neutral framework

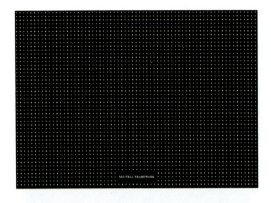

Fig. 4   The compact footprint

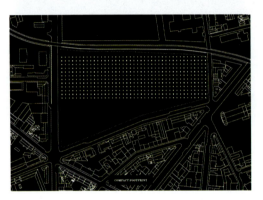

ble circulation. It is thus possible to distinguish the flows and isolate them if necessary (in a COVID crisis, for example) both vertically and horizontally. This principle, which is more costly because it requires more surface area, provides greater flexibility and versatility for the operation of the entire hospital (s. fig. 7).

The care units can then be arranged. They are all identical, allowing the caregivers to move from one department to another without losing their reference points (s. fig. 8).

Their compactness is also a deliberate choice. The main aim is to reduce travel time from one department to another, or within a department itself, from the nurses' station to the room. The number of steps taken by the nursing staff is reduced, and the energy and time spent in the corridors is time they can now spend with the patients.

The boundary between each unit is flexible and very easily adjustable. Alone or grouped by 2, 3 or 4, they can accommodate more or less important functions. The same level can be a part of the technical platform with operating theatres as well as a series of wards or consultation units (s. fig. 9).

Fig. 5   The Invariants

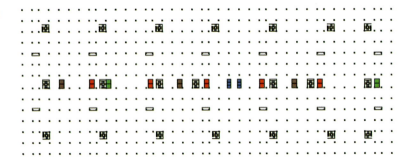

3 Hôpital Universitaire Saint-Ouen Grand Paris Nord

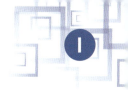

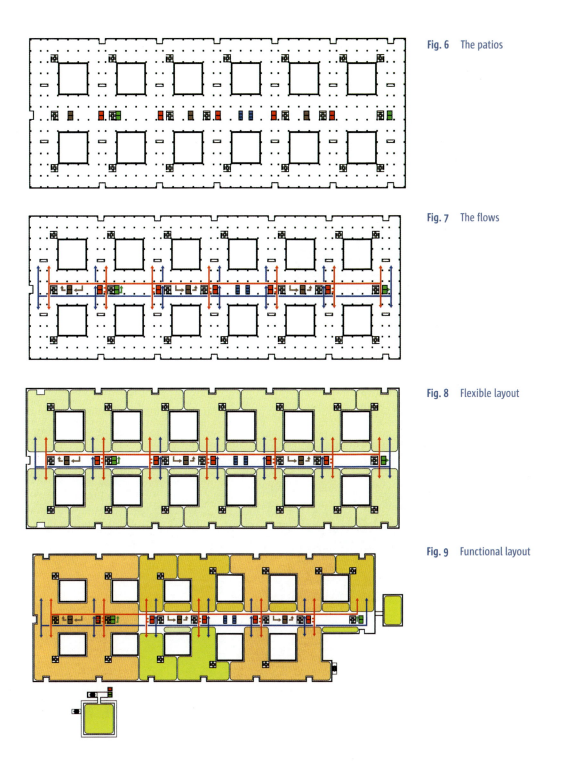

Fig. 6 The patios

Fig. 7 The flows

Fig. 8 Flexible layout

Fig. 9 Functional layout

I Flexible Frameworks

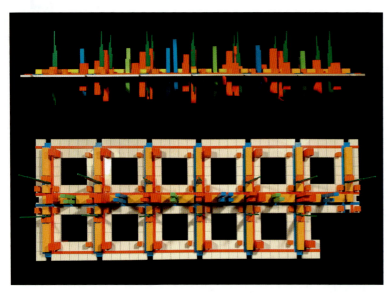

Fig. 10   Model of the large floorplan with all technical facilities

The presented model shows the principle of stratification and superimposition of these generic platforms. It also illustrates the three-dimensional development of the concept, creating an environment in which interior and exterior spaces, care areas and living areas are combined. The structure of this hospital offers a great porosity between its own world and the world around it (s. fig. 10 and 12).

The HUSOGPN, an icon of 21st century healthcare, will be a cutting-edge medical infrastructure, both human and efficient, ideally designed to meet the growing needs of the Paris metropolis in the decades to come.

Building a hospital today is about making change happen, and the HUSOGPN is emblematic of this. Staff numbers, patients and their conditions, techniques and needs are con-

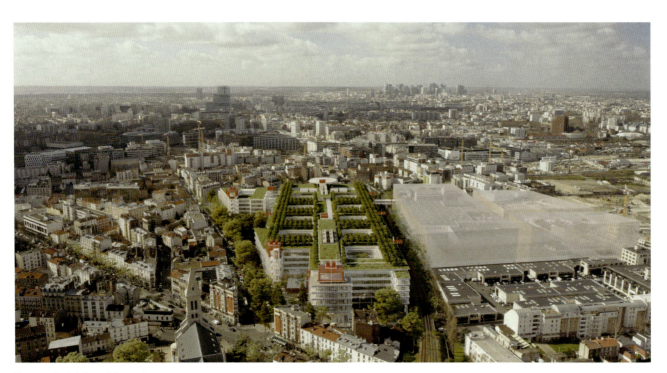

Fig. 11   Aerial view of the project

stantly changing. Designed to perpetuate the inconstant, the HUSOGPN embraces flexibility as a philosophy by remaining a permanent part of the city without ever ceasing to mutate or adapt (s. fig. 11).

The site

The site is located in Saint Ouen, a suburb of the first ring, north of Paris. At the end of the 19th century, a steam engine factory was located here, which was later transformed into a car factory and then a PSA factory. A monolith covering 35 hectares, the factory is an urban enclave that breaks away from the surrounding suburban plot of land (s. fig. 13 and 14).

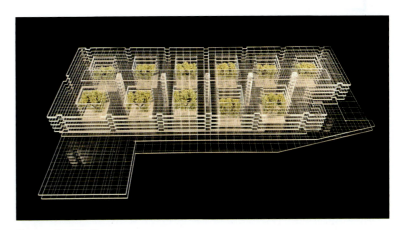

Fig. 12 Stratification

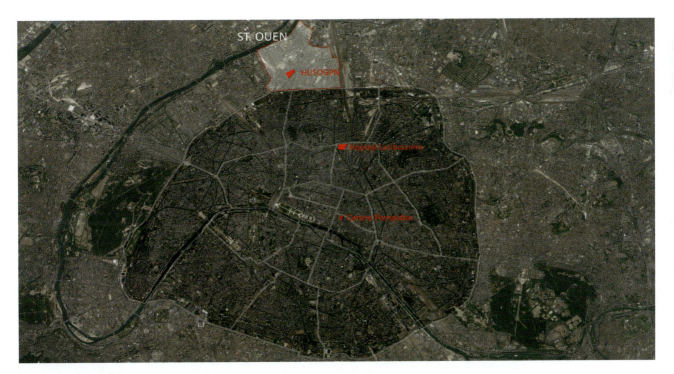

Fig. 13 Google aerial view

I Flexible Frameworks

Openness to the City

Despite the size of the programme, we wanted to make the new hospital a building that dialogues harmoniously with the city. Backing onto the railway tracks to the north, it opens onto a garden to the south, called an urban forest, which harmonises the scale of this large facility with the scale of the city. While guaranteeing the necessary privacy, the ground floors, partially double height, will be transparent to ensure the permeability of the hospital with the public space. A large forecourt invites the public to enter the building (s. fig. 15).

We have deliberately limited the height of the building to twenty-eight metres and fragmented the facades by means of gaps and "satellites." These accommodate specific functions and services such as the maternity unit and doctors' offices, making them clearly identifiable volumes on the scale of the surrounding buildings. Staircases, balconies, and satellites enliven the building's volumetry (s. fig. 16 and 17).

Fig. 14 Aerial view of the PSA site

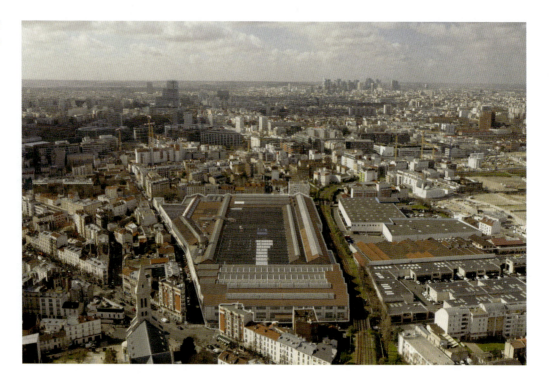

3 Hôpital Universitaire Saint-Ouen Grand Paris Nord

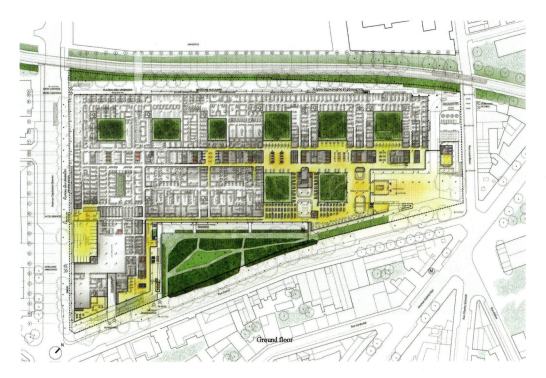

Fig. 15   Plan of the ground floor

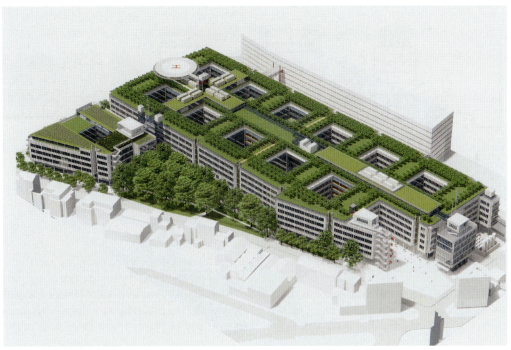

Fig. 16   Fragmentation

I Flexible Frameworks

Fig. 17 Fragments

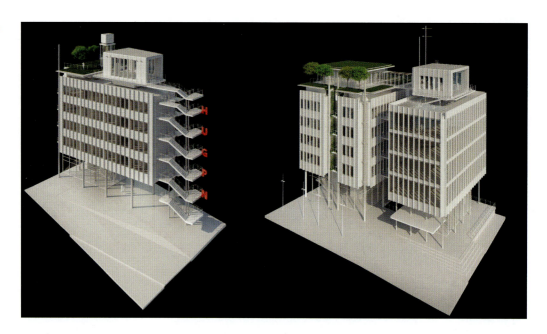

Fig. 18 Section

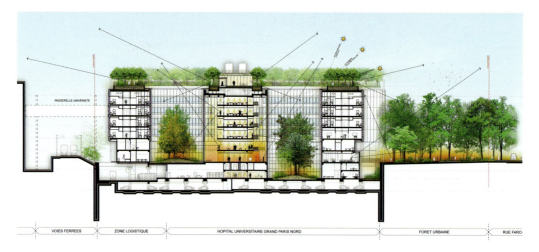

The vegetation

A factor of well-being, with recognised therapeutic virtues, vegetation is at the heart of the project. It is developed in three forms: the urban forest on the ground floor, the patios within the building and the roof garden (s. fig. 18).

Developed by our landscape designer Michel Desvignes, the urban forest will cover 2.5 hectares. It will be planted with large trees in the

3 Hôpital Universitaire Saint-Ouen Grand Paris Nord

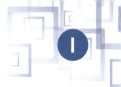

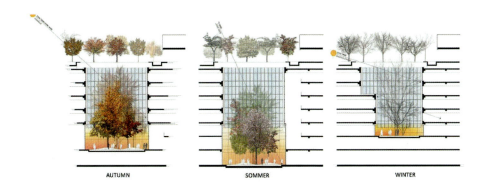

Fig. 19 Design of the patios

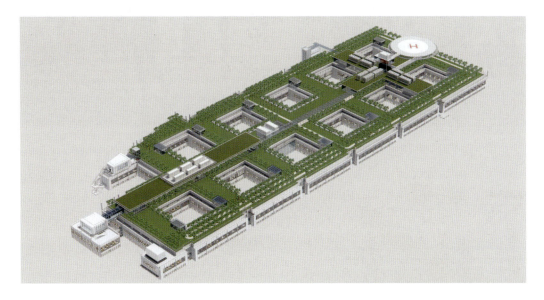

Fig. 20 Roof garden

open air that will provide shade and coolness in summer. A link between the hospital and the city, it will be a particularly pleasant and friendly place.

The patios will welcome nature within the building (in the heart of the building). Large in size (21 m x 21 m), they will punctuate the paths and provide breathing space. Planted with local or even endemic species, they will be composed in different ways, and will help to find one's way around the hospital. The plants will be carefully chosen to show the variation of the seasons, thus ensuring a constant link with the passing of time and the outside world (s. fig. 19).

The roof garden will cover 15,000 m². It will be a place of rest and breathing for medical staff, patients and visitors. It will offer a view of the city, a restaurant, common areas for staff

I Flexible Frameworks

Fig. 21 Perspective entrance hall

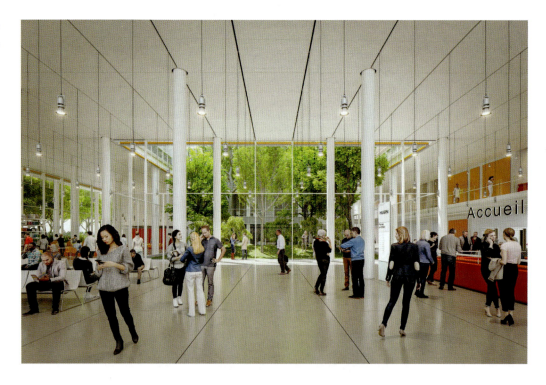

and also care areas such as a sports course and therapeutic gardens for patients (s. fig. 20).

Natural light

Like vegetation, natural light plays a major role in the healing of patients and the well-being of staff. We have been very careful to ensure that it penetrates the building as widely as possible. The patios have been designed to bring light down to the lower levels, and the two entrance halls are largely glazed and double height (s. fig. 21). The patients' rooms are equipped with three large bay windows. The windowsills have been lowered to allow patients to see outside from their beds (s. fig. 22).

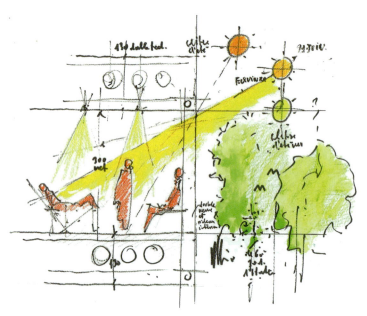

Fig. 22 Sketch Renzo Piano Chambre

Jérôme Brunet

Brunet Saunier & Associés
Paris
France

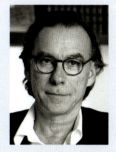

Jérôme Brunet, DPLG Architect, founded Brunet Saunier Architecture in 1981 with Eric Saunier. Together, they received the Albums de la Jeune Architecture award in 1982. In more than 30 years, Brunet Saunier Architecture has built an important body of work consisting mainly of large public facilities of all kinds, initially cultural and then hospital facilities, with a series of large facilities erected in recent years across France and Europe. Nearly twenty years of hospital design have enabled the practice to build up a solid expertise in the field of health care and to offer a transversal view, both sensitive and scientific, of the cultural variations and practices of care. Open to the international scene and familiar with large-scale projects. The practice delivered the extension of the University Hospital of Geneva in Switzerland in 2016, the Spital Limmattal of Zurich in 2018, the Jules Bordet Institute of Brussels in 2022 and the Trama Center of Helsinki in Finland in 2022. The practice is currently directing the Grand Paris Nord University Hospital.

In 2023, Brunet Saunier Architecture becomes Brunet Saunier & Associés. Four new partners (Clément Billaquois, Franck Courari, Garcie de Navailles and Hugo Viellard) joined the management of the agency at the end of 2022. The new team intends to consolidate a common vision of the project, based on a demanding and systemic approach, and to provide new responses to the major technical and environmental challenges of our time.

Thorsten Sahlmann

RPBW
Renzo Piano Building Workshop
Paris
France

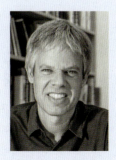

Thorsten Sahlmann graduated in architecture from the Braunschweig University in Germany and from the École nationale supérieure d'architecture of Lyon, France. Between 1991 and 2001, he worked at Helmut Riemann Architekten in Lübeck, Germany, and at Architecture Studio in Paris. Thorsten joined RPBW Architects at the end of 2001. He first worked on the renovation and expansion of the Morgan Library in New York, and on a private house project in Aspen, USA. He then worked on an office tower project for the Intesa Sanpaolo bank in Turin, Italy. He became an Associate in 2010 and was subsequently in charge of significant projects: the creation of a film research centre for the Jérôme Seydoux Pathé Foundation in Paris (2006–2014) and, more recently, the Parkapartments & Parkhotel Am Belvedere residences and hotel facility in Vienna, Austria (2013–2019). He is currently the Associate in charge of the new hospital project "Hôpital Universitaire Grand Paris Nord" in France (2020–2028).

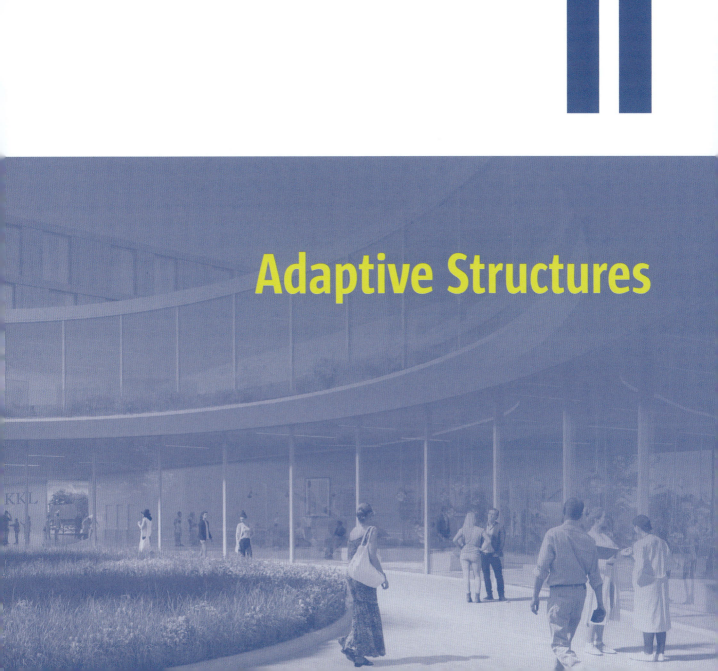

II

Adaptive Structures

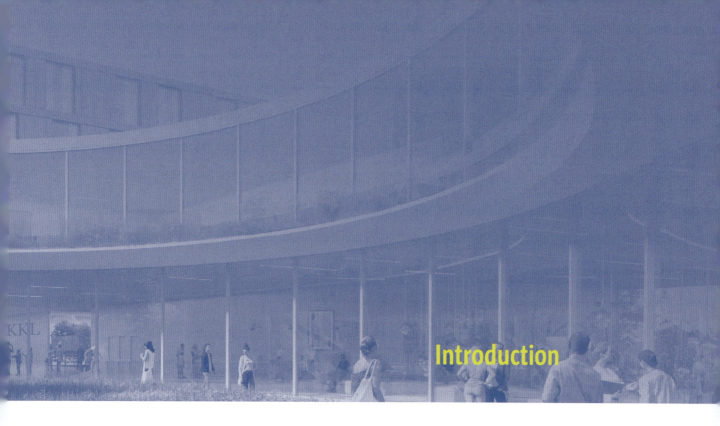

Introduction

Medicine has developed rapidly, even exponentially, since the 1970s—in just one professional generation. Above all, the doctor-patient relationship and the associated processes have changed significantly. Whereas the hospital bed used to be at the centre of medicine—the doctor came to the patient—today the hospital bed appears to function only as a parking space for the application of medicine—the patients are brought to the doctor. This reversed dynamic is a key factor in the planning of today's hospitals.

Architecture must take account of this dynamic in the health care sector. It influences several aspects that have a decisive impact on hospital processes, such as the question of single or multi-bed rooms.

Meanwhile, the construction industry has changed just as rapidly. An industry of seemingly limitless concrete resources is now faced with a health care sector that has to look for new resource-saving and recyclable options to make construction projects sustainable and fit for the future. Modular solutions are at the top of the agenda for current construction projects in response to these needs.

The following contributions examine the question of architectural solutions for adapting to rapid change in the health care sector from three very different perspectives: Nirit Pilosof shares insights from architectural research on adaptable virtual and physical spaces, Frank Jensen reports on innovative concepts of modular building technology and Reinier de Graaf presents a vision of an ideal architectural type for a future-proof hospital.

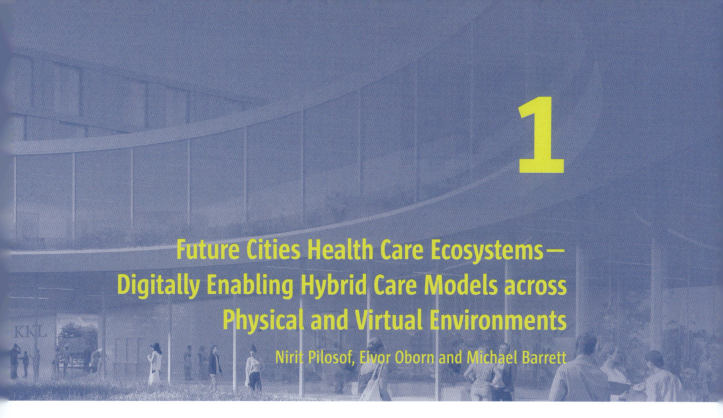

1

Future Cities Health Care Ecosystems—Digitally Enabling Hybrid Care Models across Physical and Virtual Environments

Nirit Pilosof, Eivor Oborn and Michael Barrett

Hospitals are being transformed into health care ecosystems. The notion of housing the sick in isolated facilities is being replaced by the concept of a "City of Health", an environment that promotes health and provides care at the place of living within the local community. This transformation was catalysed by the COVID-19 pandemic, which highlighted the shortcomings of existing hospital facilities and accelerated the development of digital health and remote care to connect across diverse built environments. When health care systems were challenged to prevent contamination and control hospitals' occupancy, innovations in telemedicine technologies, robotics, and AI systems provided an alternative of remote care and home hospitalisation. New hybrid models have evolved to integrate care pathways multiplied by the mode of delivery—physical or virtual—and the location of care—at the hospital, the community, or the patient home. Though hybrid models accelerate the flexibility of the health care system and provide personalised service through multiple options, the growing complexity challenges both the patient and the health care provider to control the operations and choose the best care pathway. We investigate the development of health care ecosystems in the use of telemedicine technologies for service innovation and integration of care between hospital and home, drawing on the case study of Sheba Medical Center and Sheba BEYOND, the first virtual hospital in Israel. We conclude by highlighting the potential for the development and use of Digital Twins in integrating the data of users, services, and environments to improve efficiency through real-time analytics and prediction models to support the design of the evolving health care ecosystem.

Introduction: Towards Digitally Enabled Health Care Ecosystems

The dramatic growth of digital health during COVID has accelerated opportunities to transform how health care is provided and where it is delivered. Emerging digital technologies, including remote patient monitoring, telehealth, and AI-based predictive diagnostics, have boosted the shift towards hospital-at-home services that can be scaled for improved service provisioning (Oborn et al. 2020). Recent estimates are that, by 2025, up to $265 billion worth of care services, representing up to 25 percent of the total cost of care, for Medicare fee-for-service (FFS) and Medicare Advantage (MA) beneficiaries in the US could shift from traditional facilities to the home (Bestsennyy et al. 2022). The shift of health care services from the hospital to the home and the community, enhanced by remote care integrating physical and virtual spaces, is transforming the concept of a hospital into a digitally enabled health care ecosystem (s. fig. 1).

The hospital, envisioned as a "House for the Sick", is gradually developing into a "City of Health" incorporating health promotion, continuity of care, and medical treatment. Hippocrates' vision that "The function of protecting and developing health must rank even above that of restoring it when it is impaired" (Adams 1981) is revisited by the development of digital technologies supporting health and care across

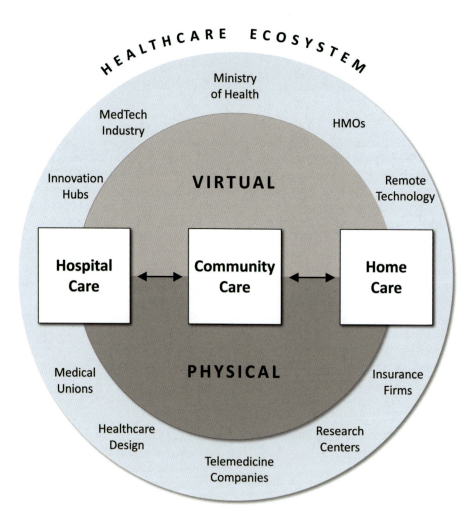

Fig. 1 The digitally enabled health care ecosystem facilitates the integration of physical and virtual care across hospitals, community-based services, and home care

the built environment. The new model of the health care ecosystem is shifting the paradigm away from providing care in a medical facility, a building with a physical location, dominated by an in-person meeting at a specific time. The health care ecosystem promotes health and care in diverse locations, both physical and virtual, in synchronous or asynchronous meetings, moving beyond the limitations of place and time. This paradigm shift requires adjustments in processes, regulations, reimbursements, business models, and collaboration initiatives from all the stakeholders involved in the health care ecosystem (Li et al. 2021; Oborn et al. 2021; Pilosof et al. 2021b; Wiedner et al. 2017).

Studies show the potential for new models of care across the health care ecosystem. Home hospitalisation, for example, can reduce costs, health care use, and readmissions, while increasing physical activity compared with conventional hospital care (Levine et al. 2020). Beneficial mechanisms include continuity of care, the power and familiarity of the home, and streamlined logistics. Patients who decline home hospital care most often lack social support at home and cite safety and the ease of remaining in the hospital as the main reasons for their decision (Levine et al. 2021a). Optimising home hospital for diverse patients and their clinicians needs to facilitate better informed discussions of the risks, benefits, and alternative service pathways from the traditional hospital (Levine et al. 2021b). The challenge is to compare and contrast different situations of care and to allow increased flexibility in selecting across various models of care. For this purpose, the system should strive to provide the right balance between hospital, community, and home care and between in-person and remote care, as complementary hybrid models and not a replacement of one service by the other.

Hypothesis: New Hybrid Models of Care

The transformation of hospitals towards a health care ecosystem accelerated through increased adoption of digital technologies during the COVID-19 pandemic. The pandemic highlighted the shortcomings of existing hospital facilities and enhanced the growth of digital health and remote care. The shift of health care services from the hospital to the home and the community, supported by remote care technologies and community-based services, led to new hybrid models of care integrating physical and virtual environments. Reinforced by the diverse stakeholders of the health care ecosystem, hybrid models of physical and virtual care hold the potential to enhance the flexibility of health care systems and provide personalised services for patients, families, and caregivers.

Case Study: Sheba BEYOND Virtual Medical Centre

Sheba Medical Center (MC) in Israel, with its ARC Innovation Centre, accelerated the use of telemedicine technologies for remote care for inpatient and outpatient care during the COVID-19 crisis. The hospital developed new models of care, including inpatient telemedicine to treat COVID-19 patients remotely within the hospital intensive care unit, internal medicine unit, and acute psychiatric unit to prevent contamination and reserve protective equipment (Oborn et al. 2021; Pilosof et al. 2021a; Pilosof et al. 2021b). The first virtual hospital in Israel, Sheba BEYOND, launched in 2021, extended this model, and developed hybrid programs for home hospitalisation. The programs led to the design of medical units with physical and virtual beds, which allowed for inpatient hospital-care with remote home-care based on patients' medical conditions and personal preferences. We see these developments as a bold move to-

II Adaptive Structures

wards leveraging a digitally enabled ecosystem strategy approach involving new hybrid models of care.

Our research, ongoing from June 2020, is based on qualitative semi-structured interviews across the Israeli health care ecosystem. The interviews include the management of Sheba MC and Sheba BEYOND, medical staff from the hospital and the Health Maintenance Organizations (HMO), IT directors, Telemedicine and Medtech organisations, architects, and policymakers at the Israeli Ministry of Health. The thematic qualitative data analysis, based on principles of naturalistic inquiry (Lincoln and Guba 1985) and a grounded approach to conceptual development (Golden-Biddle and Locke 2007), was adopted to identify emerging themes from the interviews and observations.

Results: Hybrid Care Models across Physical and Virtual Environments

Sheba MC and Sheba BEYOND, its virtual arm for remote care, developed new hybrid models of care based on a collaboration between the hospital, the HMOs' community-based care services, and the support of the Israeli Ministry of Health. The partnership between the hospital and the community services was possible only after changing regulations and reimbursement models by the Ministry of Health to promote telemedicine adoption. The dramatic increase in digital health fuelled the development and implementation of medical devices and remote technologies and allowed ongoing experimentation and testing of novel business models. The service of home hospitalisation, for example, is provided by expert doctors at the hospital with nurses from the community-based HMOs using telemedicine technologies for remote monitoring, diagnostics, and communication.

The hybrid models of care are defined by the mode of delivery, either physical or virtual, and by the location of care, either at the hospital or at the patient's home. This results in four main care pathways: (1) inpatient hospitalisation, (2) home hospitalisation, (3) inpatient telemedicine, and (4) tele-home hospitalisation (s. fig. 2).

1. **Inpatient hospitalisation—physical care at the hospital:** Traditional inpatient hospitalisation, involving bedside care by a professional medical and nursing team with medical equip-

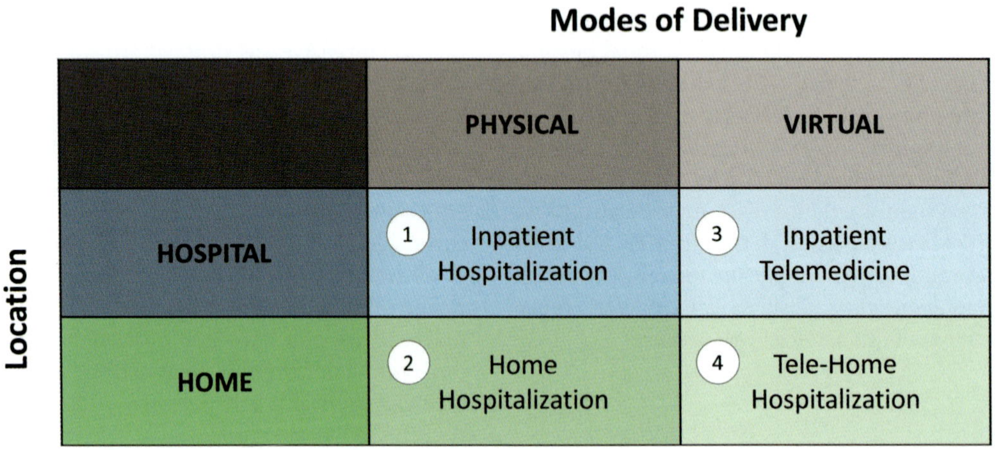

Fig. 2 Matrix of care pathways multiplied by the mode of delivery— physical or virtual, and the location of care—at the hospital or the patient home supported by community care

ment and expert support, is commonly considered the best option for critical acute patients. Although many procedures can only be performed at the hospital, inpatient care holds risks of secondary infections, delirium, falling, and physical and mental deterioration.
2. **Home hospitalisation – physical care at the patient's home**: Home hospitalisation, the relocation of care from the hospital to the patient's home, changes many aspects of care, including the patient–caregiver relationship and the family's role and involvement. The HMOs' community-based services become more central in facilitating maintenance and enhancing personal relations, mostly by nurses and local doctors. The patient's home environment often also contributes to caring by promoting comfort and minimising stress. However, this pathway is best suited for medically simpler issues that do not require advanced technologies for diagnostic purposes or direct observation by specialists.
3. **Inpatient telemedicine – virtual care at the hospital**: Inpatient telemedicine was developed during the COVID-19 crisis to provide a solution that avoids physical contact with infected patients, which significantly increases the risk of transmission and the need to quarantine exposed health care workers. The new model evolved from the electronic intensive care unit and showed potential beyond COVID to augment safety, particularly for patients who are more distant from care staff and control rooms and in circumstances of staff shortage and high occupancy rates. Although virtual care can enhance care, it also can compromise the patient's privacy and sense of control.
4. **Tele-home hospitalisation – virtual care at the patient home**: Tele-home hospitalisation was developed to maintain care during the COVID-19 crisis. Telemedicine technologies allow the medical team to care remotely for patients hospitalised at home when they are unable to accept or prefer to avoid hospital or home visits due to the risk of infections. Monitoring and supervision of patients by virtual technologies allow specialist supervision of ongoing treatment and enhance continuity of care with objective data about the patient's condition during and between encounters rather than relying on patient self-report. If the patients' condition deteriorates, they have direct access back to the hospital ward without going through the Emergency Department. However, virtual care requires the users to have technological abilities and the system to provide ongoing support.

Discussion: Flexibility across the Health Care Ecosystem

The Sheba MC study revealed the transformation process of the hospital within the evolving health care ecosystem in Israel. Although the transformation is at a preliminary stage of development, including pilots and reconfiguration of programs, it indicates a shift towards a new era of hybrid models of care. The study indicates the dependencies between the various stakeholders in the health care ecosystem and the need to collaborate, develop innovation processes, and facilitate new strategies for engagement. Understanding the stakeholders' perspectives, the needs of patients and caregivers, and the culture and roles of organisations, including competition and trust issues, is essential for advancing and scaling the new models of care.

The study demonstrates how hybrid models integrating physical and virtual environments, enabled by telemedicine technologies, foster flexibility in providing care services. Planning for change and flexibility has always been a

II Adaptive Structures

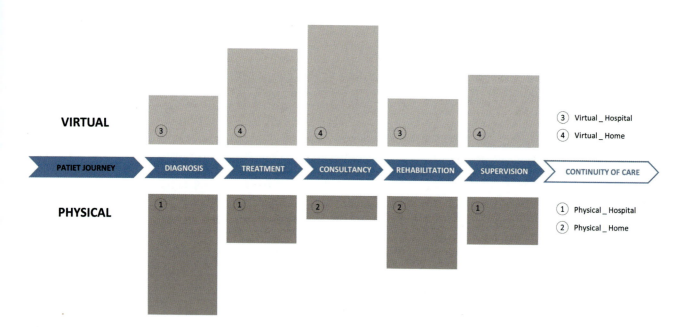

Fig. 3 Example of combinations of service modes across a patient journey (the authors; adapted from CADRE HKS, 2018)

major challenge in health care design (Pilosof 2005; Pilosof 2020). Yet, in most cases, the requirement was conceived as being only for the architecture of the building. For this reason, hospitals are often described as functionally complex and subject to frequent change over time, posing the most difficult design challenges in contemporary architecture (Hamilton 2021; Kendall 2018). COVID tested the flexibility of organisations to adapt and innovate, resulting in increased flexibility beyond the hospital to the wider ecosystem, allowing digital resilience in times of crisis.

This flexibility supports personalised patient care throughout the various phases of the patient journey, including diagnosis, treatment, and rehabilitation. Figure 3 shows the choice of care pathway available at each phase of the journey—physical care or virtual care and the location of care at the hospital or home. This choice of care provision, whether determined by the medical staff or the patients and their families, can enhance the quality of care, healing processes, human experience, and the efficiency of organisations. However, these emergent and multiplicative sets of options add to the complexity of the health care system, leaving the caregivers, the patients, and their families with a constant need to choose the best care pathway (s. fig. 3).

Conclusion: The Future Health Care Ecosystem

The future health care ecosystem holds the potential to accelerate flexibility and provide personalised service with multiple options of care. Yet, the growing complexity will challenge both patients and health care providers to control operations and choose the optimal care pathway in each case. Changing the paradigm of hospitals from providing medical treatment in designated buildings to "Cities of Health" promoting health and care in diverse physical and virtual environments call for new approaches in architecture and health care design that will support this challenge. How can architectural design go beyond focusing on designated buildings to include the inter-relationship of diverse spaces and enable the transition to the new era of digital health?

Taking inspiration from medicine, which has made significant advances moving from Evidence-based Medicine (EBM) to predictive, preventive, and personalised medicine, architecture needs to move from Evidence-based Design (EBD) to an architecture that enables predictive, responsive, and personalised places for health and care. Yet, developing an architectural design of digitally enabled health ecosystems requires the integration of digital innovation with place-making of physical and virtual environments. This development can benefit from using Digital Twins to improve operational control and patient experience (Croatti et al. 2020). Integrating the data of users, services, and environments—physical and virtual—can improve efficiency through real-time analytics and prediction models and support the design of evolving future cities' health care ecosystems.

Dr. Nirit Pilosof's presentation at the ENAH conference in March 2022 in Berlin led to the publication of a chapter in the book Future Cities—City Futures: Emerging Voices for the [(Post-)Pandemic] City, *edited by Christian Veddeler, Joran Kuijper, Michal Gath Morad, and Iris van der Wal. The book, including the chapter "Future Cities Healthcare Ecosystems: Digitally Enabling Hybrid Care Models across Physical and Virtual Environments" was published by TU Delft OPEN Publishing in April 2023.* DOI: 10.34641/mg.55

Bibliography

Adams F (1981) The genuine works of Hippocrates. William Wood & Co New York

Bestsennyy O, Chmielewski M, Koffel A, Shah A (2022) From facility to home: How health care could shift by 2025 (Issue February, p. 1–11). URL: https://www.mckinsey.com/industries/health care-systems-and-services/our-insights/from-facility-to-home-how-health care-could-shift-by-2025 (accessed August 8, 2023)

Croatti A, Gabellini M, Montagna S, Ricci A (2020) On the Integration of Agents and Digital Twins in health care. Journal of Medical Systems 44(9), 161. DOI: 10.1007/s10916-020-01623-5

Golden-Biddle K, Locke K (2007) Composing Qualitative Research. In Composing Qualitative Research. SAGE Publications, Inc. DOI: 10.4135/9781412983709

Hamilton DK (2021) Differential Obsolescence and Strategic Flexibility. Health Environments Research and Design Journal 14(4), 35–42. DOI: 10.1177/19375867211037960

HKS Center for Advanced Design Research and Evaluation (2018) CLINIC 20XX: Designing for an ever-changing present, the United Kingdom patient survey. URL: https://www.cadreresearch.org/projects/clinic-20xx (accessed August 8, 2023)

Kendall S (2018) Health care Architecture as Infrastructure: Open Building in Practice. In: Kendall S (ed.) Health care Architecture as Infrastructure. Routledge London. DOI: 10.4324/9781351256407

Levine DM, Ouchi K, Blanchfield B, Saenz A, Burke K, Paz M, Diamond K, Pu CT, Schnipper JL (2020) Hospital-level care at home for acutely ill adults a randomized controlled trial. Annals of Internal Medicine 172(2), 77–85. DOI: 10.7326/M19-0600

Levine DM, Paz M, Burke K, Schnipper JL (2021a) Predictors and Reasons Why Patients Decline to Participate in Home Hospital: a Mixed Methods Analysis of a Randomized Controlled Trial. Journal of General Internal Medicine 37(2), 327–331. DOI: 10.1007/s11606-021-06833-2

Levine DM, Pian J, Mahendrakumar K, Patel A, Saenz A, Schnipper JL (2021b) Hospital-Level Care at Home for Acutely Ill Adults: a Qualitative Evaluation of a Randomized Controlled Trial. Journal of General Internal Medicine 36(7), 1965–1973. DOI: 10.1007/s11606-020-06416-7

Li J-PO, Thomas AAP, Kilduff CLS, Logeswaran A, Ramessur R, Jaselsky A, Sim DA, Hay GR, Thomas PBM. (2021). Safety of video-based telemedicine compared to in-person triage in emergency ophthalmology during COVID-19. EClinicalMedicine 34, 100818. DOI: 10.1016/j.eclinm.2021.10088

Lincoln YS, Guba EG (1985) Naturalistic Inquiry. Sage Publications Newbury Park

Oborn E, Barrett MI, Barrett DAS (2020) Beware of the pendulum swing: how leaders can sustain rapid technology innovation beyond the COVID-19 crisis. BMJ Leader, leader-2020-000304. DOI: 10.1136/leader-2020-000304

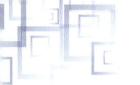

II Adaptive Structures

Oborn E, Pilosof NP, Hinings B, Zimlichman E (2021) Institutional logics and innovation in times of crisis: Telemedicine as digital "PPE." Information and Organization 31(1), 100340. DOI: 10.1016/j.infoandorg.2021.100340

Pilosof NP (2005) Planning for Change: Hospital Design Theories in Practice. AIA Academy Journal 8, 13–20

Pilosof NP (2020) Building for Change: Comparative Case Study of Hospital Architecture. HERD: Health Environments Research & Design Journal, 193758672092702. DOI: 10.1177/1937586720927026

Pilosof NP, Barrett M, Oborn E, Barkai G, Pessach IM, Zimlichman E (2021a) Telemedicine Implementation in COVID-19 ICU: Balancing Physical and Virtual Forms of Visibility. Health Environments Research and Design Journal 14(3), 34–48. DOI: 10.1177/19375867211009225

Pilosof NP, Barrett M, Oborn E, Barkai G, Pessach IM, Zimlichman E (2021b) Inpatient telemedicine and new models of care during covid-19: Hospital design strategies to enhance patient and staff safety. International Journal of Environmental Research and Public Health 18(16), 8391. DOI: 10.3390/ijerph18168391

Wiedner R, Barrett M, Oborn E (2017) The emergence of change in unexpected places: Resourcing across organizational practices in strategic change. Academy of Management Journal 60(3), 823–854. DOI: 10.5465/amj.2014.0474

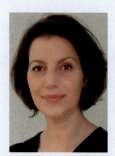

Dr. Nirit Pilosof

Tel Aviv University
Coller School of Management
Tel Aviv
Israel

Nirit Pilosof is an architect and researcher exploring the intersection of health care, technology, and architecture. She is a Faculty Member at the Coller School of Management, Tel Aviv University, and an Associate of Cambridge Judge Business School (CJBS) at the University of Cambridge in the UK. She is also Head of Research in Innovation and Transformation at Sheba Medical Centre, and the Executive Member of Israel at the International Union of Architects (UIA) Public Health Group. Nirit Pilosof holds a PhD from the Technion – Israel Institute of Technology, a Post-Professional M. Arch from McGill University, and an Evidence-Based Design Accreditation and Certification (EDAC) from the Center for Health Design in the USA. She has won international awards, including the prestigious American Institute of Architects (AIA) Academy of Architects for Health award, the American Hospital Association (AHA) graduate fellowship, the McGill Graduate fellowship, and the Azrieli Foundation fellowship.

1 Future Cities Health Care Ecosystems — Digitally Enabling Hybrid Care Models across Physical and Virtual Environments

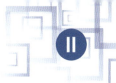

Prof. Eivor Oborn

Warwick Business School
Coventry
United Kingdom

Eivor Oborn is a Professor of Healthcare Management in the area of Innovation and Organisational Change at Warwick Business School, UK. She earned her PhD at Cambridge Judge Business School, the University of Cambridge in 2006, and is currently an honorary Fellow at Cambridge Judge Business School and Fellow at the Cambridge Digital Innovation Centre (CDI). Eivor is Senior Editor at Information Systems Research and has published work in leading journals, including Academy of Management Journal, Organization Science, Information Systems Research and MISQ. Her scholarship has won numerous awards including best published paper from American Medical Informatics Association (AMIA) and Academy of Management (AOM). Her research interests span the fields of healthcare, online communities, digital innovation & ICTs, as well as entrepreneurship in ecosystem contexts. She teaches in the area of Change Management, Strategic Health Leadership and Corporate Entrepreneurship.

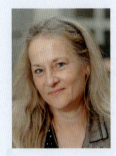

Prof. Michael Barrett

Cambridge Judge Business School
Cambridge
United Kingdom

Michael Barrett is a Professor of Information Systems & Innovation Studies, Director of research at Cambridge Judge Business School (CJBS), Director of Cambridge Digital Innovation, and a Distinguished Visiting Professor of Innovation at the Stockholm School of Economics. Michael Barrett published in many top-tier IS (Information Systems) and Organisation journals, and has won several best paper awards at EGOS and the Academy of Management (AOM) and award winning teaching cases. He is the Editor-in-Chief of the *Information & Organization journal* and is on the Advisory Board of the *Journal of the Association of Information Systems*. He has contributed to articles in *The Economist*, *The Times* and *The Financial Post*, and has served as an external examiner at Oxford University, the University of Edinburgh and the London School of Economics. Professor Barrett has served as a stream research lead for the Cambridge Digital Built Britain, on the Steering Board of the Cambridge Service Alliance and as a member of the Management Executive Group of the knowledge translation research group Collaborations for Leadership in Applied Health Research and Care (CLAHRC).

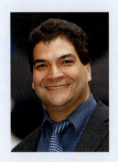

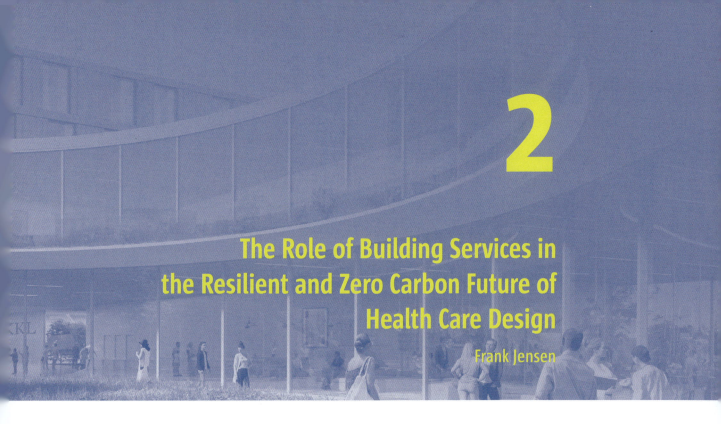

2

The Role of Building Services in the Resilient and Zero Carbon Future of Health Care Design

Frank Jensen

The demands on the quality and robustness of the building services in health care are ever increasing. This drives significant investments in floor space, systems and operations.

However, there is a cost-effective alternative to the traditional system design. An alternative where the focus is not on providing flexibility through robustness, but instead on acceptance of the uncertainty that is inherent in any prediction of the future. In this alternative paradigm, the building services systems are designed for repeatability and resilience, thereby reducing the overall cost of the systems and also the wider hospital facility.

Robust customisation

Hospital facilities are large capital investments designed to last fifty years or more. They have therefore always presented planners with the thankless challenge of predicting both the future needs of the population served and the technological development in the decades to come.

To meet this challenge, planners, architects and engineers have traditionally been future-proofing buildings through generalisation, flexibility and elasticity:

- Generalisation is the ability of a building to meet changing functional requirements *without the need to adapt* the building's structure, facade or building services. An example of this is the change of an office space into a single-bed room.
- Flexibility is the ability of the building to meet changing functional requirements *through changes* to the building's structure, facade or building services, i.e. the possibility of making changes to the building with minimal costs and disruption.

- Elasticity is the ability of the building to allow expansion and/or reduction in the useable floor area through extensions and subdivision of the building.

The above approach is not unique to the design of hospital facilities as similar challenges are also encountered within infrastructure projects, IT-development and military procurement.

Critics argue that the above approach leads planners to falsely believe that they can sufficiently predict future functional requirements and therefore can plan and specify for all relevant eventualities, and ultimately procure future-proof health care facilities.

However, this approach instead most often leads to monolithic and customised projects where redundancy upon redundancy (over-specification) are built into the project to ensure sufficient robustness to meet future demands. The results are most often delays, budget overruns and expensive operations.

Resilient modularity

Alternative successful approaches to the design of complex projects have been building momentum over the last decades and are being promoted by business leaders and academics.

One approach promotes repeatable modularisation of the project as it is planned and constructed, thereby obtaining speed in planning and execution as well as modular replicability (Flyvbjerg 2021). Speed ensures that what is being built is not yet obsolete at the time of the opening, while modular replicability allows for early experimentation and continuous learning throughout design and construction processes.

A second approach is focused on understanding that projects often become complicated and over-specified because of a perceived need for a completely integrated design. It is argued that the development of a basic platform should be decoupled from the development of the supporting systems that provide actual capabilities (Greenert 2012). Through such a decoupling, the development of the platform can be both accelerated and simplified, while individual supporting systems can be continuously developed and upgraded independently of the platform itself. Thus, the classical over-specification and robustness can be replaced by a simpler and more resilient framework or project.

Novel paradigm

For the New Odense University Hospital, a novel paradigm for building services was developed based on the two novel approaches proposed above. Initially, the key driver was value engineering, but during its development other key motivations were discovered as the clear advantages of going from a robust custom design to a resilient modular design became apparent for the client, architects, engineers and hospital planners.

Early research for the paradigm focused on the value engineering opportunities of reducing the floor area needed for the air handling units (AHUs). This is because any reduction herein will also reduce the surrounding floor area needed for circulation, facades and partition walls, making it a key driver in an increased or decreased ratio for gross-to-net floor area.

It was investigated how the overall planning and design of the hospital would be affected if either far fewer and larger AHUs or far more, smaller AHUs were to be implemented. The latter was easily preferable as the many smaller units could be placed in the voids above the suspended ceilings in both primary and secondary rooms, thereby completely eliminating the need for floor area for these small AHUs.

The reason that there are useable voids above the suspended ceiling is that the gross height of

2 The Role of Building Services in the Resilient and Zero Carbon Future of Health Care Design

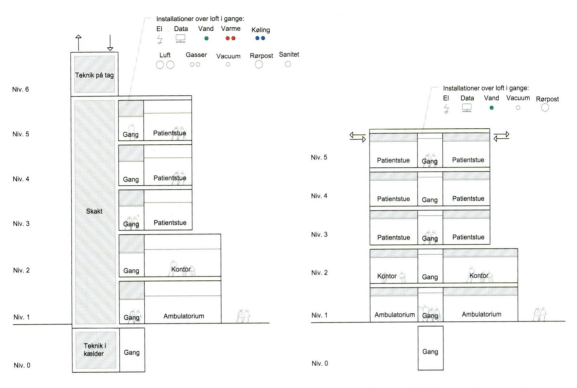

Fig. 1 A novel paradigm for building services with a focus on simplification, modularity and space utilisation. The key driver is mechanical units located above the ceiling in individual rooms

individual floors are most often determined by the need for building services routing in narrow corridor spaces. Hence, any removal of air ducting would also reduce the gross height of the building (s. fig. 1).

Based on this early research and findings it was clear that by going from bespoke AHUs with their associated ducting to smaller standardised AHUs located above the ceiling in the individual rooms would be beneficial for the project. Not only from an initial investment perspective, but also because the planning of the hospital would not be constrained by maximum duct lengths and shaft positions, thereby allowing a simpler and easier to modularise layout.

Future changes in functional requirements would also be simpler to implement, as there would be no interdependency of rooms and functions through shared AHUs. And finally, benefits of technological developments in both building services and medico-technical equipment would become much easier to harvest. This is because upgrades to AHUs would no longer be a construction project to be planned and executed but instead a simple upgrade or replacement of a small standardised unit.

Desk study

The next round of development of the paradigm was focused on establishing references, validation and discovering further benefits. Taking reference from the International Space Station

Fig. 2 Surgical ward cross section of corridor with mechanical units (one for fresh air and three for recirculation) placed in every room

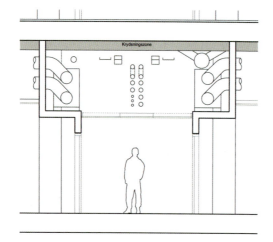

Fig. 3 Bed ward cross section of corridor with mechanical units placed decentralised in every room

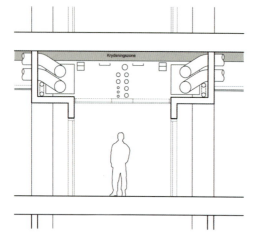

and many military applications, it was clear that all building service systems—both mechanical and electrical—could be modularised, and each individual room-sized module could be made to be near-independent of its neighbour as long as each module was serviced by an infrastructure of sewage, data, electrical and cold water supply.

The paradigm was thereafter extended to include a number of system solutions, which are all rarely used in hospital design—all with the aim of simplifying the bespoke infrastructure and instead decentralising and standardising all the supporting systems, thereby treating them more as equipment rather than building parts.

Vacuum toilets were integrated, providing reduced water use, improved hygiene and horizontal routing. Electrical busbars gave increased flexibility. Electrical point-of-use water heaters and/or filters reduced energy and water consumption while increasing water quality. Furthermore, decentralised waterless sprinkler systems and point-of-use storage of gases were investigated.

With all major building services systems having been found capable of supporting both modularisation and decoupling of the supporting systems from the building infrastructure through extensive use of point-of-use components, it was time to investigate the buildability of the paradigm.

A number of reference projects and suppliers were visited. These visits and interviews uncovered the possibility of applying modern methods of construction within the developing paradigm and hence potential for improvements in quality, lower risks and better cost management.

The final part of the desk study was to ensure the small AHUs were capable of providing both comfort and hygiene ventilation. The initial step was to engage with stakeholders to get (as a first in Denmark) permission to use air recirculation in operating rooms (ORs) and wherever else relevant. This reduced the amount of fresh air the units needed to supply by a factor of four. Built on this, it was decided that for ORs three recirculation AHUs could be used for hygiene ventilation and a single standard AHU could be used for comfort ventilation i.e. fresh air.

By omitting the major air ducts, all intakes and exhausts would have to penetrate the facade at the point-of-use. Using CFD simulations it was found that the external air dilution, due

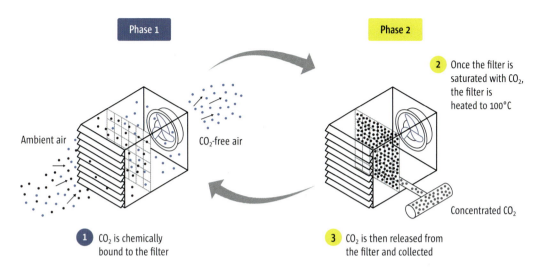

Fig. 4 The global climate crisis is leading to a cap on lifetime CO_2-emissions from buildings as well as Direct Air Carbon Capture (DACC) technologies (Beuttler et al. 2019; available in Open Access CC BY 4.0)

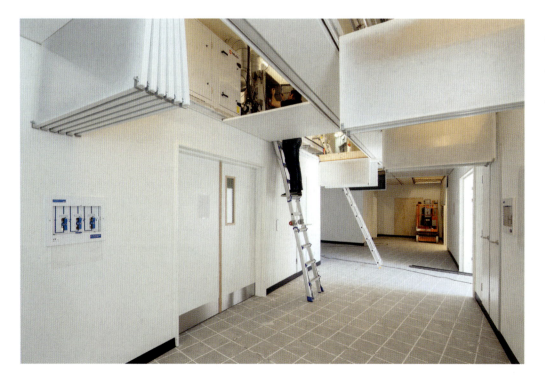

Fig. 5 Photo from the mock-up corridor demonstrating access to the mechanical units placed on a shelf above the rooms

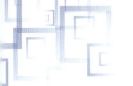

to high exhaust velocity in combination with standard air filters, could reduce the cross-contamination to acceptable (very low) levels.

The final improvement to the AHUs was the integration of a reversible heat pump into the comfort ventilation unit. This permitted all heating and cooling pipes to be omitted from the building infrastructure and the heating/cooling of the building to be fully electrified and thus sourced renewably.

The result of the continuing development was thus that across bed wards, office spaces and ORs a small standardised AHU for comfort ventilation had been developed integrating all needs for filters, heating, cooling and airflow (s. fig. 2 and 3). Supplemented with an equally standardised recirculation AHU, it had been shown that nearly all of the ventilation needs of the entire university hospital could be met by a modular, safe and efficient approach. An approach that reduced the consequences of single unit failure and would also support a plug'n'play strategy for increased preventive maintenance.

Proof-of concept

A full-scale prototype of the comfort AHU was built and tested with the purpose of validating particularly the heating and cooling capabilities. The unit was built using standard components including a rotary heat exchange unit and a reversible heat pump.

Building on this AHU prototype, a more extensive mock-up was designed and built inside the hospital's innovation centre (s. fig. 5). This successful mock-up included a small number of typical rooms such as a corridor, OR, bed, office and toilet and demonstrated the advantages in positioning the AHUs on a corridor shelf above the rooms, allowing for easy lift access and safe working conditions for facility management.

Future development

The still-developing climate crisis will cause further uncertainty in the design of hospitals, particularly large developments. In Denmark, the government has already implemented stringent rules for permitted carbon emissions throughout a building's life cycle. From 2023 until 2029 the current levels of emissions are required to be nearly halved and the trend is expected to continue downwards thereafter.

Going forward, any masterplan for a health care facility will be faced with an accelerating pace of development within the sustainability space. In fact, it is expected that there will be near-continuous changes to the legal framework, technologies, energy costs, carbon taxes etc. The importance of modularity and resilience has never been higher.

And maybe, just maybe, such resilient hospitals will have an important role to play in saving not only patients but also the planet. Being modular and thus allowing for rapid experimentation, it would be a logical next step to start looking at Building Integrated Carbon Capture (BICC) through the integration of standard carbon dioxide scrubbers in the AHUs (s. fig. 4). This is a well-known technology. Coupled with hospitals' high rates of air change and the possibility of on-site regeneration of the filters, BICC promises not to only make the hospital life-time carbon neutral, but possibly carbon negative, thereby saving not only its patients but also the planet!

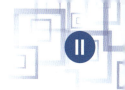

Bibliography

Beuttler C, Charles L, Wurzbacher J (2019) The Role of Direct Air Capture in Mitigation of Anthropogenic Greenhouse Gas Emissions. Frontiers in Climate 1. DOI: 10. 10.3389/fclim.2019.00010

Flyvbjerg B (2021) Make Megaprojects More Modular. Harvard Business Review. November-December Issue, 58–63

Greenert JW (2012) Payloads over Platforms: Charting a New Course U.S. Naval Institute Proceedings 138(7), 16–23

Dr. Frank Jensen

Søren Jensen Rådgivende Ingeniørfirma
Aarhus
Denmark

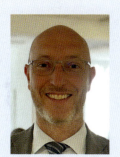

Frank Jensen is the third-generation head of the family business of Søren Jensen Consulting Engineers and leads its investments in companies related to sustainable construction through carbon accounting, SMART Buildings, and upcycled, recycled and organic construction materials.

He is trained in both mechanical and structural engineering as well as in architecture and holds a PhD in the design of adaptable structures. He has led the engineering design for hospitals in excess of one million square metres and has executed a number of high-profile projects with architects such as Frank Gehry, Kengo Kuma, Snøhetta, Dorte Mandrup and others.

Frank Jensen is engaged in several advisory roles spanning from research to social housing. Through his engagements, he aims to take responsibility for and reduce the significant environmental impact of the construction industry. Søren Jensen has, under his leadership, been certified as a B Corp and has pledged to make its projects zero-carbon by 2030.

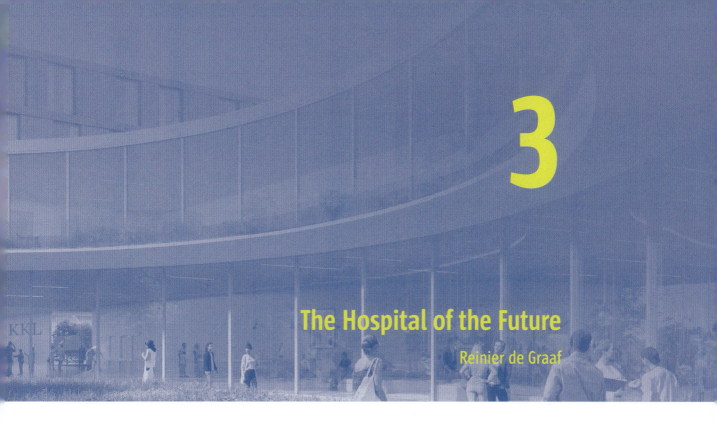

3

The Hospital of the Future

Reinier de Graaf

Al Daayan Health District: A Picture Series from the Presentation by Reinier de Graaf, OMA

How to respond to the ever-changing demands of the health care system? The author calls for a radical rethink in the construction of hospitals towards flexible and adaptable structures. He presented his vision for a future-proof health facility in the design of the Al Daayan Health District, situated on a 1.3 million square metre site on the outskirts of Doha, Qatar. Its description reads like a manifesto:

> "Can we imagine a different way to build hospitals? Instead of building high, what if the hospital were a low-rise structure? Conceived not as a building, but as a system made up of modules, incorporating gardens where nature can be enjoyed by patients and staff. A limited number of elements accommodates an array of functions—a structure that can be scaled up or down, yet remains operational at all times, adaptable to changing demands, organised around a network of flows. This is the hospital of the future. The hospital of the future builds itself; it maximises the potentials of automation and 3D-printing and uses its waste as a resource. The hospital of the future produces what it consumes: its energy, its food, its medicine." (OMA: The Future of the Hospital www.oma.com/news/oma-reinier-de-graaf-and-squint-opera-release-video-of-new-hospital-prototype)

II Adaptive Structures

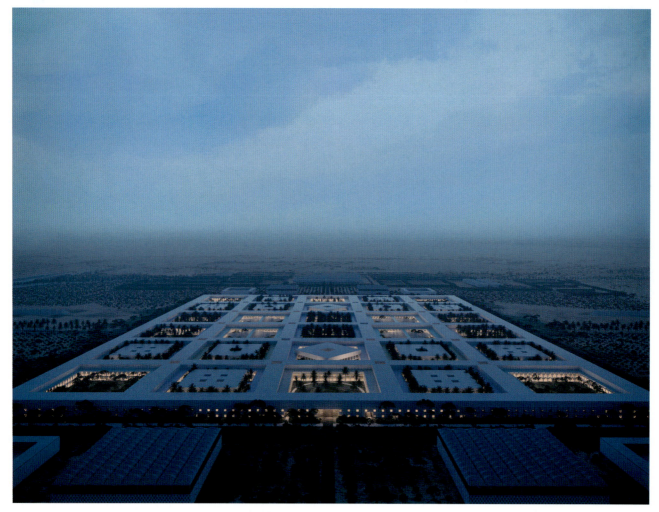

Fig. 1 The flat building structure of the Al Daayan Health District is organised in modules and encompasses 30 courtyards. It consists of only two storeys (s. fig. 2 and 3) and prioritises ground-level access to the gardens (s. fig. 4) for all 1,200 patient beds, while the examination and treatment rooms are located on the first floor. An underground level connects all areas through a system of tunnels for automatic transport of goods. Outpatient care units are integrated into the courtyards as freestanding "villas" (s. fig. 5 and 6) © HMC

3 The Hospital of the Future

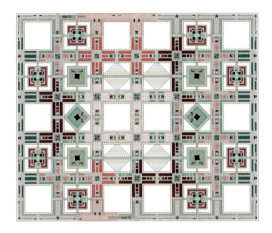

Fig. 2 First floor © HMC

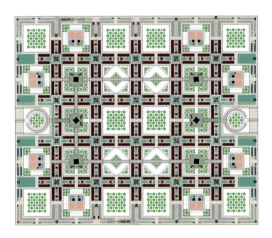

Fig. 3 Ground floor © HMC

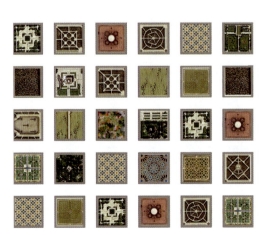

Fig. 4 Gardens and patios © HMC

II Adaptive Structures

Fig. 5 Modules © HMC

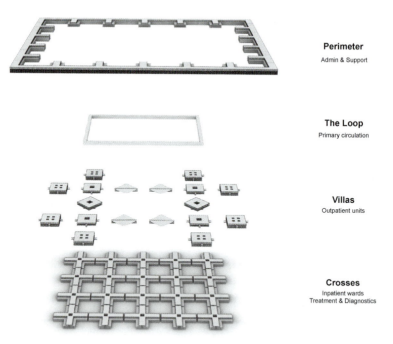

Perimeter
Admin & Support

The Loop
Primary circulation

Villas
Outpatient units

Crosses
Inpatient wards
Treatment & Diagnostics

Fig. 6 "Cross" module and "Villa" © HMC

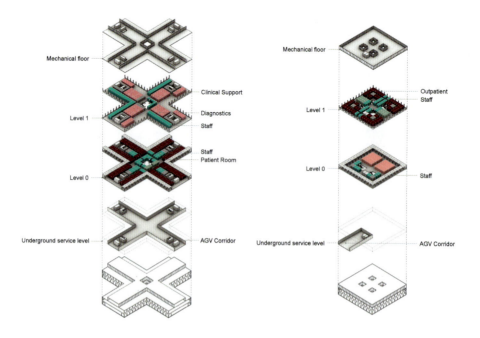

58

3 The Hospital of the Future

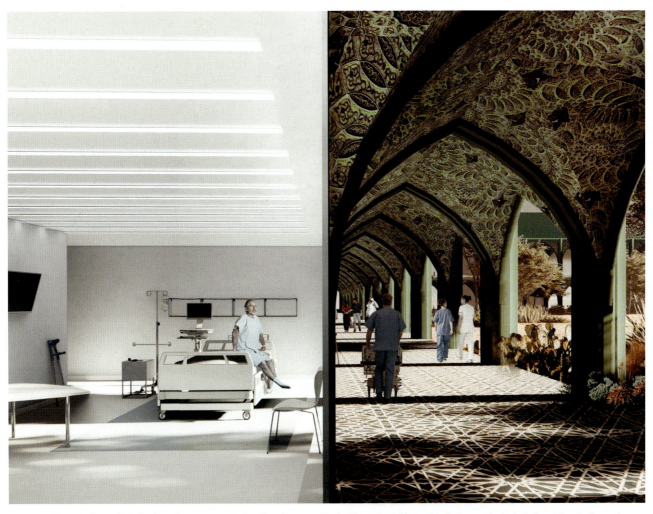

Fig. 7 Galleries in front of the bed wards represent the interface between the inside and outside worlds, between the technical and the sterile on the one side, and the natural and the emotional on the other. © HMC

II Adaptive Structures

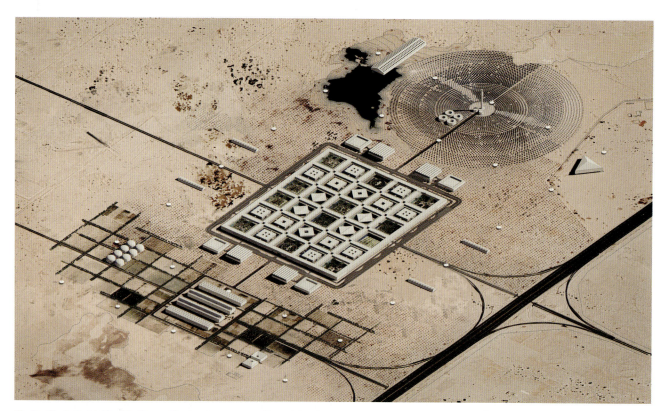

Fig. 8 The industrial health city—resilient, autonomous, self-sustaining © HMC

Fig. 9 Like an autarkic industrial site, the clinic building is supplemented by infrastructure and research hubs, including a high-tech farm for food and medicine production, a solar energy park, and a 3D printing centre, where the ornaments for the courtyard facades will be developed. © HMC

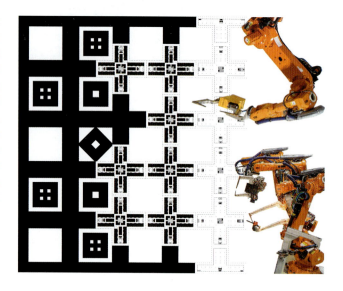

3 The Hospital of the Future

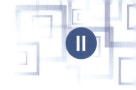

Team

Reinier de Graaf (Partner-in-Charge), Kaveh Dabiri (Project Architect), Alex De Jong (Project Manager), Pablo Antuna Molina, Claudio Araya, Bozar Ben-Zeev, Joana Cidade, Benedetta Gatti, Eve Hocheng, Sofia Hosszufalussy, Hanna Jankowska, Tijmen Klone, Marina Kounavi, Hans Larsson, Roza Matveeva, Geert Reitsma, Alex Retegan, Silvia Sandor, Elisa Versari, Arthur Wong

Collaborators

- Masterplan Engineering: BuroHappold
- Landscape Architect: Michel Desvigne Paysagiste
- Clinical Architect: Henning Larsen Architects
- Healthcare Planning: ETL
- Wayfinding: Spaceagency
- Cost Adviser: De Leeuw Group
- Stakeholder Management: Engineering Consultants Group

Client

Hamad Medical Corporation

Image Copyright HMC

The images may not be passed to any third parties without further permission. No part of the work may be reproduced or utilised in any form or by any means, electronic or mechanical, including photocopying, recording or by any information storage retrieval system, without permission in writing from HMC.

Reinier de Graaf

Office for Metropolitan Architecture (OMA)
Rotterdam
The Netherlands

Reinier de Graaf is a Dutch architect and writer. He is a partner in the Office for Metropolitan Architecture (OMA) and the co-founder of its think-tank, AMO. He is the author of *Four Walls and a Roof: The Complex Nature of a Simple Profession* (Harvard University Press 2017), *The Masterplan* (Archis 2021), and *Architect, verb* (Verso 2023).

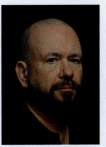

by Adrienne Norman, © OMA

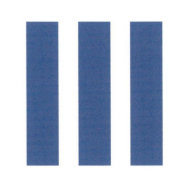

Fix — Recover — Prevent

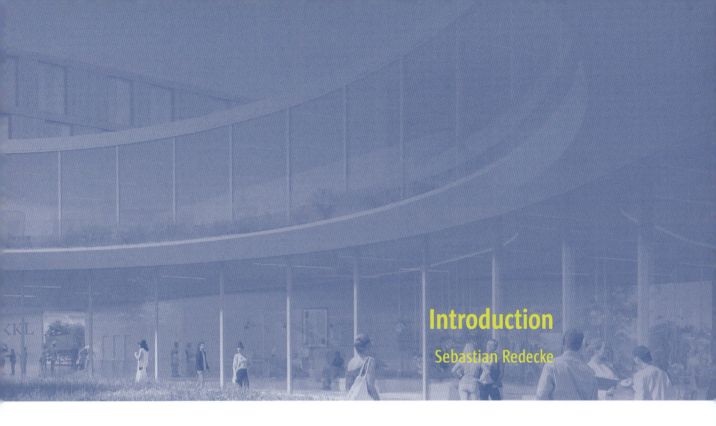

Introduction

Sebastian Redecke

Fix—recover—prevent. Fix in a hospital, recover at home, prevent everywhere. Health care services are to be seen as a whole, as a package with many differentiations and optimally organised with partners. How should planning offices, from architects to specialist engineers, react to this conceptual complexity? What concrete tasks do they have to deal with?

New ways have to be found in the organisation of hospitals, and far beyond, for the entire health care system. In this context, structural management, taking into account intensive interaction, is crucial for care, treatment and individual processes. Especially in the context of shortened stays, better coordinated outpatient care or therapy is important, and also requires separate planning of treatment centres that guarantee good care in rural areas. Much attention should be paid to this interlocking, instead of persisting with partial responsibilities and individual players, which patients usually have to endure with negative consequences.

What is needed is a fast organisation with problem-free data transfer.

My hope, however, is that the trend "doctors as service providers, patients as customers", in a hospital trimmed to efficiency and a health system trimmed to efficiency, will not at some point have a demonstrably detrimental effect, as it leads to great dissatisfaction and can thus even influence the healing process. A proper balance is therefore very important here. In addition, a new, strongly interconnected overall concept of treatment and care raises the question for planning: which essential influencing factors can be derived, not only from the pandemic but also from today's form of society with its significant changes in living together, in order to inform the conception of a hospital of the future?

In any case, flexible structural solutions and quick changeover will have to be incorporated into planning specifications. However, transportable solutions are now also of greater im-

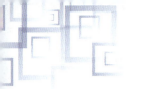

portance, especially in view of the global development in the field of health care buildings. The task for planners will increasingly be to develop concepts with mobile room modules that are relatively easy to produce, transport and equip. They form the basic framework for healthcare facilities with different tasks in different layouts, from bed wards to highly complex technical units. According to the requirements and clear objectives on site, they can also be erected on a temporary basis. It would certainly take a great deal of effort to promote such a concept internationally with all those involved at the political and planning levels. But this is the only way to take a big step towards better equipment in health care on a global level, in a way that conserves resources, reduces costs, saves time and, last but not least, is clearly effective in terms of planning.

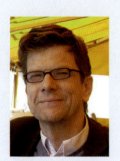

Sebastian Redecke, Dipl.-Ing. Arch.

Bauwelt
Berlin

Sebastian Redecke studied architecture at the Technische Universität Braunschweig and at the Università La Sapienza in Rome. Since 1990, he has been an editor at the architecture journal *Bauwelt* in Berlin. He is co-editor and co-author of several books on architecture and urban planning in Berlin and Paris.

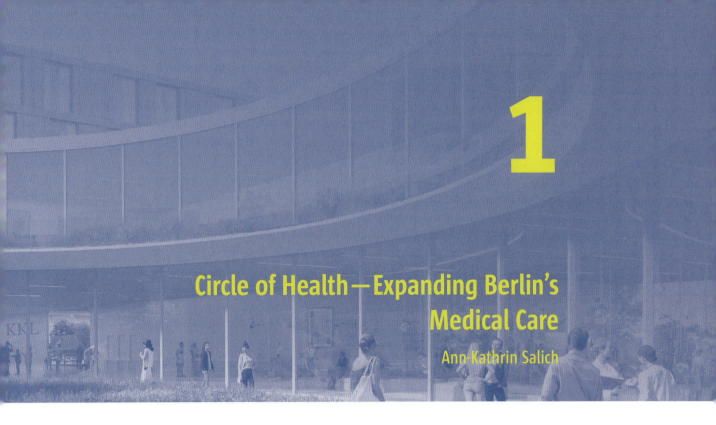

1

Circle of Health — Expanding Berlin's Medical Care

Ann-Kathrin Salich

Besides the well-known Corona pandemic, one can also recognise a worldwide "pandemic" of chronic diseases. Cardiovascular disease, cancer, diabetes mellitus, Parkinson's, depression, addiction etc. are tremendously increasing (Robert Koch-Institute 2015). In addition to the demographic change, this presents a huge future challenge for the health care sector and social system. This is because severe illnesses lead to incapacity to work, need for care, and very expensive treatment. Therefore, from a macro-economic and social point of view, one needs to think of measurements to help people stay healthy until old age. Fortunately, science has already found many factors that strongly influence the risk of getting these kinds of conditions and thus provides information on ways to prevent them. Science has proved that many illnesses are strongly linked to our living conditions, health behaviour and social status. It is proven that, for example, stress, negative dogmas, malnutrition, obesity, addiction, little physical activity, unhealthy diet, toxins, pollution, etc., all severely increase the risk of getting ill. Sadly, the health statistics of our highly urbanised society and people's health behaviour is very worrying. In Germany, 70 percent of men, over 50 percent of women and 15 percent of children are overweight (Robert Koch-Institute 2015) Only one third of Germany's population are physically active for more than two hours a week (Robert Koch-Institute 2015). Thus, it is crucial that people establish a healthy lifestyle with a balanced diet, sufficient physical activity, abstinence from any kind of drug, and with regular health checks. However, implementation can be very difficult. Additionally, the constantly changing trends and recommendations make it nearly impossible not to get confused.

So, where do we find reliable information? Where can we practice positive behaviour? Could architecture potentially help us to face this challenge?

This led me into an urban analysis of Berlin's medical facilities. I recognised that Berlin has a

III Fix—Recover—Prevent

Fig. 1   Circle of Health

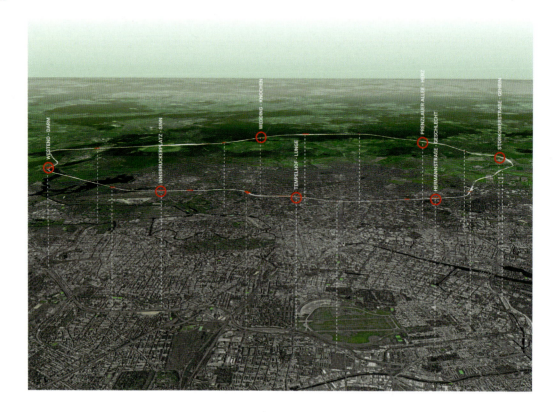

vast selection of treatment facilities, but due to their urban positions, their appearance and the medical services they offer, they are not comprehensive enough to be effective for prevention. Accordingly, I realised that Berlin needs a new typology of patient-focused prevention centres. Health centres that are located within the city, where people would regularly pass by, without needing to specifically search for them. Health centres which are compelling enough to encourage regular visits. Health centres which focus on prevention. Health centres whose architectural design already raises awareness about health topics and encourages a change in behaviour by functioning as urban hotspots.

Accordingly, I developed an architectural masterplan, specially designed for Germany's capital city, Berlin. It proposes an architectural design of modular health care centres located on the Berlin "S-Bahn Ring." The "S-Bahn Ring" is Berlin's most important and iconic public transport infrastructure. It circles Berlin's city centre, connects all railway lines, runs through most Berlin districts, and connects the inner city with its outskirts. It is highly frequented every day, all round the clock, and by a large part of Berlin's population of all social classes. Therefore, it offers great potential for confronting people with health topics.

I discovered a repetition in the way in which the stations are positioned within the urban context, which I utilised to develop a modular architecture with education, relaxation and movement sections. Each of those departments

1 Circle of Health—Expanding Berlin's Medical Care

are included into each of the seven building types, offering treatments corresponding to the typology. The placement of these buildings on the S-Bahn Ring means that all people can access each of these seven buildings and thus gain the opportunity to truly advance their health in all seven categories, offering a fully holistic approach that has never been seen before.

The result is the "Circle of Health" (s. fig. 1), making health care more inclusive, visible, and attractive within the urban landscape. Further, I developed the idea of multiple different types of health centres. Each type focuses on a different health topic, as within my medical analysis, I realised the complexity of illnesses and the impossibility of creating one building that fits all. My research led me to discover seven parts of the human body that have the most influence on health, and that their interplay offers a truly comprehensive holistic system of healing and prevention. Whereas classic medicine offers health consultation based on medical specialisations, I am allowing a different division that focuses more on the patients, their symptoms and their healing pathway. The result is the creation of seven buildings that on their own each represent a comprehensive healing modality for the chosen health topic. But in their interplay, they offer a truly comprehensive holistic system of healing and prevention.

Based on the declaration of the World Health Organization that health is "a state of complete physical, mental and social well-being and not merely the absence of disease or infirmity", (WHO n.d.) I developed a system of "four pillars of health", which consists of four sections: treatment, education, relaxation and movement. They are built into each of the seven buildings and are adjusted according to each building type and theme. The placement of these buildings on the S-Bahn Ring means that all people can access each of the seven buildings. Thus, all can gain the opportunity to truly advance their health in all seven categories.

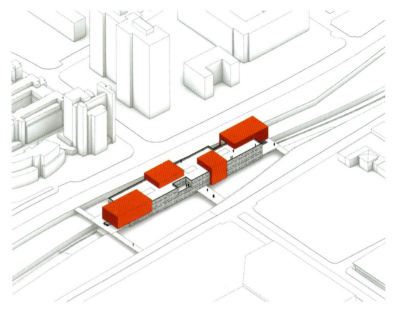

Fig. 2 Brain Building

The "Circle of Health" offers a fully holistic approach that has never been seen before.

Brain

Illnesses of the neuronal system, such as Parkinson's, dementia and MS are increasing. There are indications that stimulating your brain with cognitive training, learning new skills and interacting socially can lower your risk for these kinds of diseases (Angelucci et al. 2015; Cantarero-Prieto et al. 2018). Accordingly, the "BRAIN" building offers the opportunity to train your brain with challenges. Visitors directly enter the public playground with its multiple brain training exercises such as chess, sudoku and lyric games, which naturally are integrated into the interior design. This space encourages social interaction and activity in a daily manner, e.g. on the visitor's way back home (s. fig. 2).

III Fix—Recover—Prevent

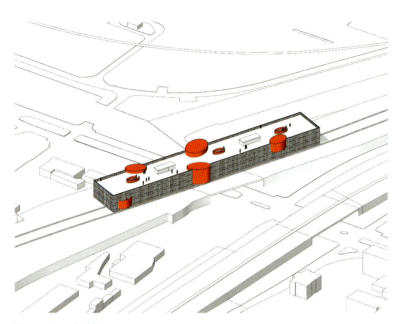

Fig. 3   Lungs Building

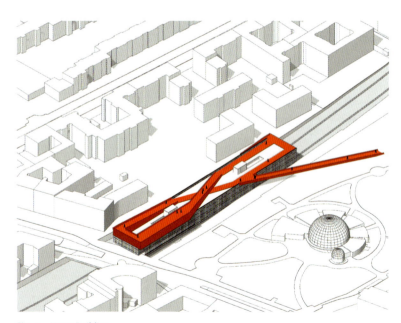

Fig. 4   Heart Building

This architectural vision was achieved using a system of "boxes in the box." All treatment departments are located in "private boxes", leaving space for the brain training playground. Each box has a clearly visible typography and an individual reception which helps with orientation in the building. Furthermore, the playground itself has a diverse and iconic design to help with orientation. This is especially crucial for those visitors who already have neuronal issues.

Lungs

Our lungs provide us with oxygen, which we need for living, 17,280 times a day, unconsciously. However, our lungs are highly underacknowledged organs. Especially in the city, our lungs are exposed to unhealthy emissions, pollutions and other chemicals. Further, we mostly sit in closed rooms with high CO_2 levels, which can produce short-time adverse reactions like headaches and fatigue but can also lead to respiratory symptoms (Singleton et al. 2017; Fisk et al. 2019).

On top of this, there are still 28 percent of German citizens who smoke (Rauschert et al. 2022). Therefore, it is highly important to give our lungs a break in order to let them recover. The "LUNGS" building aims to integrate rooms with clean air and with different temperatures and humidities to facilitate the self-healing process (s. fig. 3). This was achieved by creating multifunctional "air bubbles" which can be used for seminars or waiting rooms. They are equipped with different plant species, including those recommended by the comprehensive NASA study (Wolverton et al. 1989), to clean the air of pollution and toxic chemicals. Additionally, they can simulate different climate conditions which can strengthen your lungs (Kingsley n.d.). While the visitors are educa-

1 Circle of Health — Expanding Berlin's Medical Care

ted about respiratory health, the architecture itself simultaneously helps their lungs to recover.

Heart

Cardiovascular illnesses are currently some of the most widespread diseases. The RKI obtained data that one third of Germany's population is estimated to have high blood pressure (Robert Koch-Institute 2015). This is a huge problem because this raises the risk for heart attacks and other heart diseases tremendously. It is proven that physical exercises, especially cardiovascular training, help to lower weight and improve blood circulation which can both prevent heart-related issues (Santos et al. 2020; Tofas et al. 2019).

Accordingly, the architectural aim for the "HEART" building was to motivate its visitors to get moving and enjoy it (s. fig. 4). This was realised by implementing a huge running loop starting at street level, leading the people to enter the building, run through it, and finish on the roof. This running loop was additionally connected with an extra pathway to the local park, aiming to attract other pedestrians.

Furthermore, the functions were distributed in such a way as to emphasise the idea of walking. The building is cut into four pieces crossing each other. On the ground floor level, there is the Treatment department and the Relaxation department. Whereas the Treatment department is smoothly accessible, one needs to go to the first floor to the Movement department to access the Relaxation area. On the first floor, there is also a restaurant situated within the Education department.

Sense

An illness usually does not appear out of nowhere. Our body sends us messages to make us

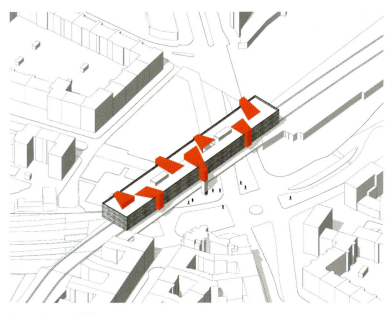

Fig. 5 Sense Building

aware of malfunctions in advance. But unfortunately, we often don't recognise these signs, or we even consciously repress them (Kolnes et al. 2012).

This is very dangerous for our health, because the earlier we identify health problems, the better we can treat them and prevent more dangerous conditions. Concerning psychological disorders, the recognition of symptoms is often the first step towards healing. Therefore, it is extraordinarily important to learn and train self-awareness and consciousness.

Accordingly, the "SENSE" building enables and facilitates self-observation and body-mind-connection by offering rooms with special atmospheres (s. fig. 5). These rooms have a funnel shape and a skylight in order to promote a focus on oneself rather than being distracted by other visuals. These rooms are kept relatively dark and sound protected so that one's senses are limited and one is inclined to go within and exclusively hear and see oneself. These rooms are equipped with minimalistic seating to as-

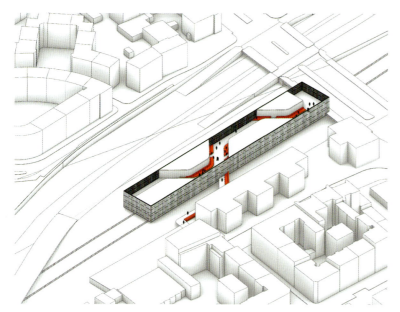

Fig. 6 Gut Building

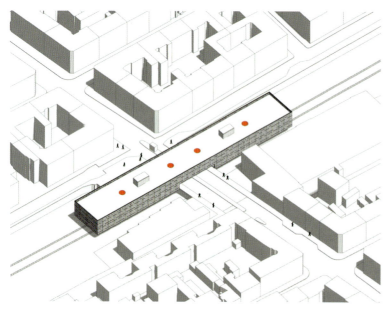

Fig. 7 Gender Building

sist in getting into deep meditations, which are shown to increase individual introspective accuracy (Fox et al. 2012).

Gut

The intestine is often called our second brain. Evolutionarily, the brain and intestine have developed out of one tissue. Nowadays the Vagus Nerve still physically connects our brain with our intestine. Therefore, our intestine can possibly influence our mind as much as our mind influences our intestine. It is proven that an unbalanced bacterial flora affects our mood negatively and that nervousness and anxiety can lead to digestion problems (Zhang et al. 2015). Therefore it is as important to feed our body with the right food as it is to practise calmness and serenity.

The problem is that our stressful and hectic daily life often makes it difficult to stay connected and calm. But data shows that it is very important to listen to our intuition, take breaks and eat slowly and deliberately. Otherwise, we tend to overeat, consume the wrong food or swallow too-large bites which can lead to obesity or illnesses (Leahy et al. 2014; Cherpak et al. 2019).

Therefore, the architectural aim of the "GUT" building was to make the visitors sit down, take a break and relax for a moment (s. fig. 6). This was achieved by installing comfortable sitting and sleeping places throughout the whole building. This building has the concept of separated departments to make the guests visit one department after another and give them the possibility to take a break in between. All medical and educational consultations happen on the ground floor level, whereas the pavilions on the roof are extensions to house multifunctio-

1 Circle of Health—Expanding Berlin's Medical Care

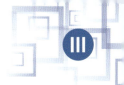

nal community and relaxation activities as well as restaurants.

Gender

A rising number of young people have issues with themselves—their look, their body shape or their gender. Advertisements, pornography and social media suggest a perfect but unrealistic image of how we should be or look, so that young people tend to be ashamed of their own natural body. Mindsets such as body-shaming and self-hate are deconstructive and dangerous because they can lead to severe mental illnesses like eating disorders, depression or self-harm, accelerating the risk of other physical illnesses (Brewis and Bruening 2018).

Therefore, it is tremendously important to start accepting and loving oneself. The architecture of the "GENDER" building aims to positively shape one's body feeling (s. fig. 7). This was realised with a delicate, curved interior. The idea was to enable the visitors to get themselves into new body positions and carefully accustom themselves to gentle touches.

Bones

Life never goes the way we expect it to. Crises naturally occur, as we have seen with the corona pandemic. An important protection factor is mental resilience. Psychological resilience is the opposite of vulnerability and helps us to feel good despite unfavourable living conditions. Research shows a strong cross-effect between mental health and physical health. It emphasises that physical activity is one of the largest contributors to better mental health (Ohrnberger et al. 2017).

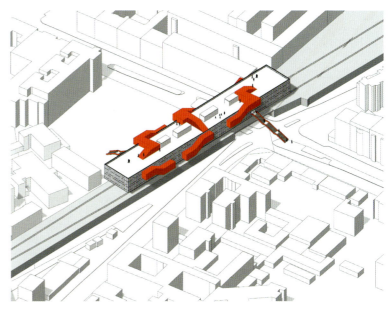

Fig. 8 Bones Building

Therefore, the "BONES" building focuses on improving mental resilience by offering physical training (s. fig. 8) This is achieved by a modular sports parkour aiming to challenge the visitors with daring obstacles. Due to its modular structure, the parkour can be adjusted to keep up the challenge in the long term. Training this ability and overcoming barriers strengthens our mental as well as our physical health tremendously. As a desired side effect, this kind of sports activity strengthens our bone structure and could potentially prevent illnesses like osteoporosis (Pinheiro et al. 2020).

This is especially important for our society, because women in particular are nowadays in great danger of getting osteoporosis (Keen and Reddivari 2023). Sport activities such as weight lifting, trampolining or stair climbing are very beneficial for osteoporosis prevention (Iwamato 2017).

Bibliography

Angelucci F et al. (2015) Cognitive training in neurodegenerative diseases: a way to boost neuroprotective molecules? Neural Regeneration Research, DOI: 10.4103/1673-5374.169608

Brewis AA, Bruening M (2018) Weight Shame, Social Connection, and Depressive Symptoms in Late Adolescence. Int J Environ Res Public Health, DOI: 10.3390/ijerph15050891

Cantarero-Prieto D et al. (2018) Social isolation and multiple chronic diseases after age 50: A European macro-regional analysis. PLoS ONE, DOI: 10.1371/journal.pone.0205062

Cherpak CE (2019) Mindful Eating: A Review Of How The Stress-Digestion-Mindfulness Triad May Modulate And Improve Gastrointestinal And Digestive Function. Integrative medicine (Encinitas, Calif.)

Fisk W et al. (2019) Do Indoor CO_2 Levels Directly Affect Perceived Air Quality, Health, or Work Performance? Ashrae Journal

Fox, KCR et al. (2012) Meditation experience predicts introspective accuracy. PLoS one, DOI: 10.1371/journal.pone.0045370

Iwamato J (2017) A role of exercise and sports in the prevention of osteoporosis. Clin Calcium 27(1)

Keen MU, Reddivari AKR (2023) Osteoporosis in Females. StatPearls

Kingsley C (n.d.) Best (And Worst) Weather For COPD. URL: https://lunginstitute.com/best-weather-for-copd/ (accessed 14 April 2023)

Kolnes L-J et al. (2012) Embodying the body in anorexia nervosa–a physiotherapeutic approach. Journal of bodywork and movement therapies, DOI: 10.1016/j.jbmt.2011.12.005

Leahy K et al. (2014) The Relationship Between Intuitive Eating and Postpartum Weight Loss. Maternal and Child Health Journal, DOI: 10.1007/s10995-017-2281-4

Ohrnberger J, Fichera E, Sutton M (2017) The relationship between physical and mental health: A mediation analysis. Social Science & Medicine. URL: https://www.sciencedirect.com/science/article/pii/S0277953617306639 (accessed 14 April 2023)

Pinheiro MB et al. (2020) Evidence on physical activity and osteoporosis prevention for people aged 65+ years: a systematic review to inform the WHO guidelines on physical activity and sedentary behaviour. Int J Behav Nutr Phys Act 17(1)

Rauschert C et al. (2022) The Use of Psychoactive Substances in Germany. Deutsches Ärzteblatt international, DOI: 10.3238/arztebl.m2022.0244

Robert Koch-Institute (2015) Health in Germany—the most important trends. Federal Health Reporting. URL: https://www.rki.de/DE/Content/Gesundheitsmonitoring/Gesundheitsberichterstattung/GBEDownloadsGiD/2015/kurzfassung_gesundheit_in_deutschland.pdf?__blob=publicationFile (accessed 14 April 2023)

Robert Koch-Institute (2015) Hoher Blutdruck: Ein Thema für alle. URL: https://edoc.rki.de/handle/176904/3138 (accessed 29 September 2023)

Santos L et al. (2020) Exercise, Cardiovascular Health, and Risk Factors for Atherosclerosis: A Narrative Review on These Complex Relationships and Caveats of Literature. Frontiers in Physiology, DOI: 10.3389/fphys.2020.00840

Singleton R et al. (2017) Housing characteristics and indoor air quality in households of Alaska Native children with chronic lung conditions. Indoor Air, DOI: 10.1111/ina.12315

Tofas T et al. (2019) Exercise-Induced Regulation of Redox Status in Cardiovascular Diseases: The Role of Exercise Training and Detraining. Antioxidants, DOI: 10.3390/antiox9010013

WHO (n.d.) Constitution. URL: https://www.who.int/about/governance/constitution (accessed 14 April 2023)

Wolverton BC, Douglas WL, Bounds K (1989) Interior landscape plants for indoor air pollution abatement(Report). NASA

Zhang Y-J et al. (2015) Impacts of Gut Bacteria on Human Health and Diseases. Int J Mol Sci 16(4)

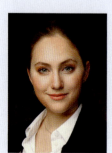

Ann-Kathrin Salich

Technische Universität Berlin

Ann-Kathrin Salich is a young architect with a passion for visionary ideas and practices. She graduated from the Technische Universität Berlin and has studied at the Technische Universität Delft and in Zurich. She works at the architectural office Nickl & Partner and teaches digital designing and modelling methods at the Leibniz University in Hannover. Her interest in health care architecture was shaped from an early age by her parents, who worked in the medical field. She aims to make a positive impact on the health care sector and its building designs. Her master's thesis "The Circle of Health—expanding Berlin's medical care" won the Charité Prize 2022 and received public attention. She has presented at the ARCH22 conference in Delft und the Healthy City Conference in London.

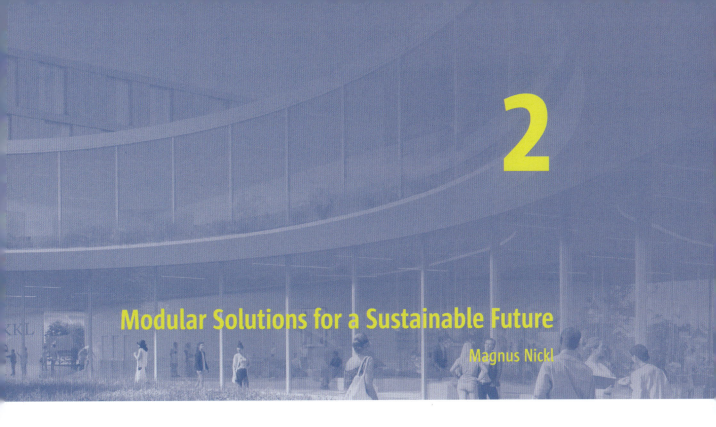

Modular Solutions for a Sustainable Future

Magnus Nickl

A transformation is underway, catalysed by a fresh perspective on health care architecture and innovative design methods. This paradigm shift is marked by a fundamental change in approach—a departure from traditional construction methods towards off-site prefabrication of architectural elements without compromising on quality. Future hospitals are envisioned as an assemblage of individual healing units, each tailored to enhance patient care.

This evolution in practice is not without purpose; it emerges in response to the pressing challenges we face. Climate change, energy supply constraints, and resource scarcity are potent drivers compelling architects to embrace modular construction techniques. The delicate balance between risks and advantages, coupled with the fluctuating dynamics of the global economy, longs for a resilient and adaptable approach to hospital design. Moreover, the changing nature of localism and mobility dynamics accentuates the urgency for architects to address issues of privilege, marginalisation, and equity within health care spaces. New responsibilities are emerging:

- the promotion of global health and well-being,
- encouraging standardisation and unity in health care infrastructure and
- tackling emerging medical dangers are the new goals.

Modular construction stands out as a solution, offering a variety of advantages. A new understanding of sustainability, with reduced material waste and increased energy efficiency, is an integral component of this eco-conscious approach. Innovation in design, strategic systems, and adaptability are key factors, allowing architects to create flexible, future-proof buildings that can seamlessly adapt to evolving needs.

Additionally, cost efficiency and fast prototype design lead to construction processes that reduce disruption to ongoing medical services. The concept of flexible partitioning not only

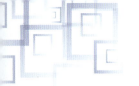

enhances space utilisation but also allows for tailored environments that adapt to diverse patient requirements, while faster occupancy and use become achievable.

In conclusion, through the integration of modular building techniques in health care architecture we enter a new era of design innovation. As architects with an understanding of global challenges and a keen sense of responsibility, we are redefining the future of health care infrastructure and shaping environments that foster healing, promote inclusivity, and aim for a healthier, more sustainable world.

Reducing risks through modular innovations

The reduction of risks lies at the core of modular design. Innovative construction methods, combined with better control and supervision of contractors' work, form the construction process. By incorporating standardised designs and precise execution, architects and engineers can significantly minimise errors and enhance accuracy. Repetitive calculations by skilled professionals further contribute to this precision, ensuring a seamless and error-free production of modules. Moreover, we ensure consistency and reliability by careful planning and creating a safer and more predictable construction environment.

Sustainability through modular layering

As a result, modular innovations introduce a concept of layering that transcends traditional boundaries. Starting from the smallest module of an architectural element, such as the intelligent wall designed for the "Health Box" project, this approach progresses seamlessly to larger structural elements. Individual units are integrated into frameworks, forming cohesive, self-sustaining volumetric units supported by a robust skeleton design. As this modular framework expands, it transforms into complete structures, flexible and adaptable, capable of accommodating a variety of uses.

In contrast to common belief, modularity isn't only confined to temporary or emergency applications. The aim is to design buildings which outlast their initial purpose. The variety in assemblage, from intricate structural elements to versatile, fully functional networks of modules, showcases longevity and adaptability. In essence, architects and engineers are not only constructing buildings made of sustainable materials; they are crafting ecosystems in which risk reduction strategies and sustainable modular layering take us a step forward.

Examples of our work

The following exemplary projects redefine the essence of "Healing Architecture" by blending functionality, sustainability, and adaptability into their architectural DNA.

Kaiser-Franz-Josef Spital, Vienna, Austria

The Kaiser-Franz-Josef Spital in Vienna, initially intended for temporary use, surpassed its intended lifespan due to its robust framework design. By integrating fully prefabricated modules into a dynamic framework, the building functions as a metabolic entity, with modules of varying lifespans contributing to its durability. The modular approach not only enabled swift construction but also ensured the building's longevity, making it a symbol of architectural resilience.

LVR Klinik Haus D, Cologne, Germany

The LVR Klinik Haus D challenges conventional hospital design: Constructed from just two modules, it allows for experimentation with different layouts and future additions. The project breaks away from traditional constraints and embraces modular flexibility (s. fig. 1–4).

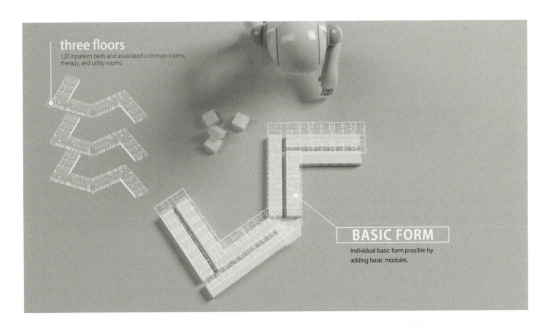

Fig. 1 Addition of the basic modules to form a care unit at LVR-Klinik Köln

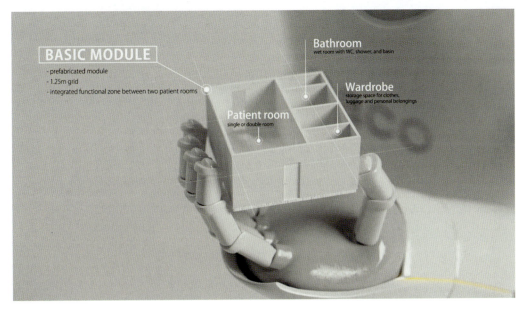

Fig. 2 Modules are prefabricated and based on a grid of 1.25 m

III Fix—Recover—Prevent

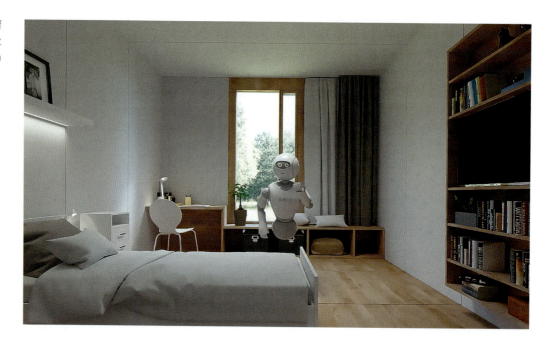

Fig. 3 Visualisation of a future patient room at LVR-Klinik Köln

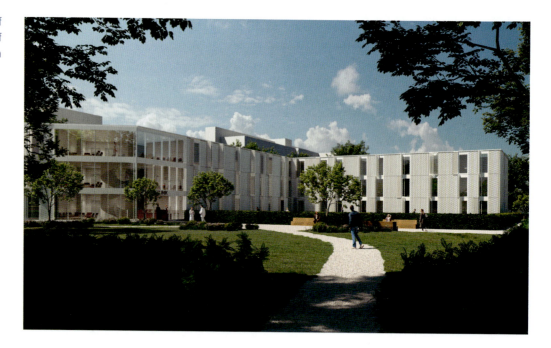

Fig. 4 Visualisation of new modular building of LVR-Klinik Köln

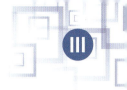

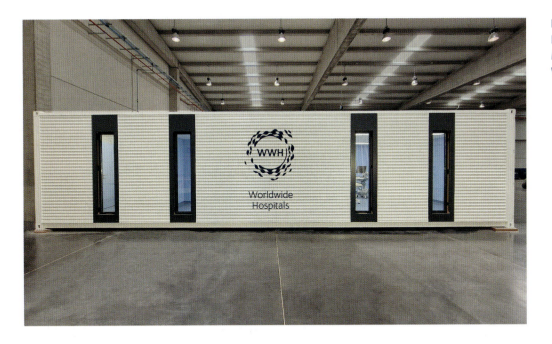

Fig. 5 Equipped 30m² High-Cube Heavy Duty Medical Module (credits: WWH)

Pocket Hospital Citra, Indah City, Indonesia

The Pocket Hospital Citra in Indah City, Indonesia, stands as a masterpiece of hybrid construction and decentralised design. Prefabricated walls and beams, strategically used to overcome challenges associated with traditional frameworks, are seamlessly integrated into the structure. The incorporation of prefabricated steel support beams, filled with lightweight concrete, provides stability and prevents issues like ceiling corrosion.

Ventilation and air handling systems are distributed across individual units. This decentralised approach not only simplifies the complex health care architecture but also enhances productivity and quality by allowing tailored, controlled workflow conditions during manufacturing.

Health Box

The Health Box project pioneers structural element design, encapsulating all mechanical, electrical, plumbing, and insulation components within prefabricated walls. By eliminating complications related to maintenance and integrating essential elements into one single architectural element, it transcends the conventional approach.

Thinking outside the box: Redefining the future of health care with hospital ships

A pioneering concept that has emerged is the utilisation of containers as building blocks. Central to this ground-breaking vision is the aim to create functional prototypes, which are

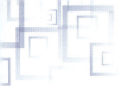

III Fix—Recover—Prevent

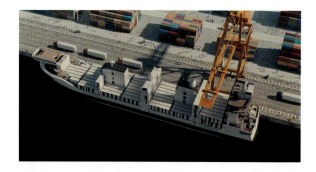

Fig. 6 Hospital ships can be ready for mission within 3 days (credits: WWH)

Fig. 7 Mock-up of the hospital ship's patient rooms

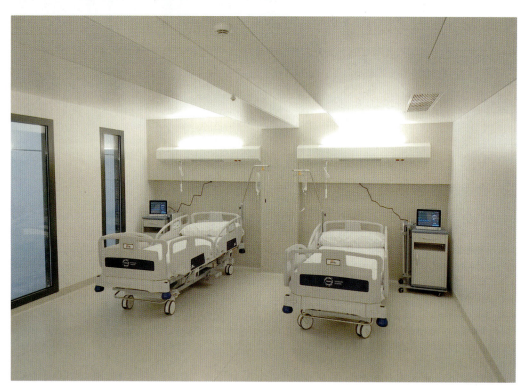

built under sustainable circumstances and can be easily assembled and transported. The decision to repurpose old containers is not only cost-effective but also underscores a commitment to sustainable practices by reducing the demand for new materials.

Furthermore, the utilisation of standardised containers offers a host of advantages, from worldwide standard sizes to optimised space usage due to efficient shipping capacities. The structure of these containers, designed for space efficiency, lays the foundation for a transforma-

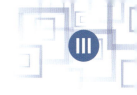

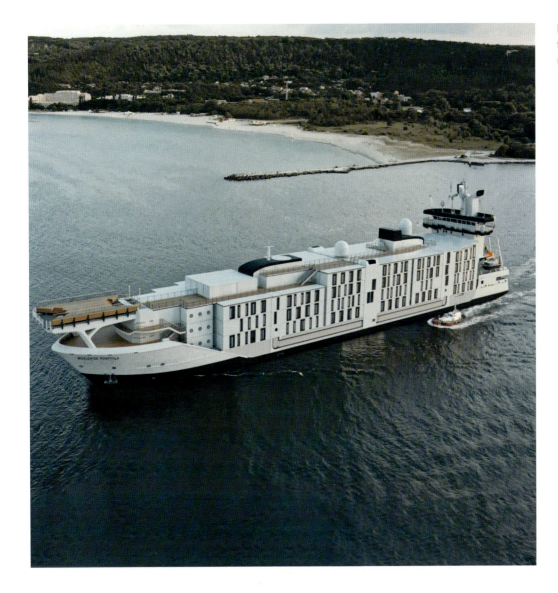

Fig. 8 Visualisation of the modular Hospital Ship (credits: WWH)

tive spatial program within confined quarters. It is possible to achieve standardised hospital typologies by forming larger intervention rooms, theatres and multi-bedroom units out of containers.

Moreover, this method is efficient from a long-term perspective since it allows flexibility, easy adaptation and modification for various purposes, and easy disassembly and reuse, ensuring that they can be reconstructed elsewhere or repurposed for multiple projects. Even in cases where modules are not reused, the design for disassembly ensures a sustainable process compared to traditional construction and demolition methods (s. fig. 5–8).

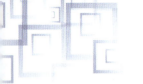

III Fix—Recover—Prevent

Envisioning the future: Long-term impacts

Looking ahead, the implementation of this approach holds the promise of long-term positive effects. Beyond immediate health care provision, these modular structures open avenues for adaptive reconfiguration, ensuring that they remain relevant and functional for evolving health care needs. By embracing these principles, architects and health care professionals are not only redefining the future of hospital spaces but also setting new standards for environmental responsibility and adaptability in health care architecture.

Thus, hospital ships become more than vessels; they transform into symbols of innovation, sustainability, and resilience, navigating the challenging seas of health care, arriving in a new era where healing environments are not confined by land but extend across oceans, reaching those in need with compassion, efficiency, and a profound commitment to a sustainable future.

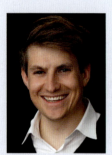

Magnus Nickl

Nickl Architekten Schweiz AG
Zurich
Switzerland

Magnus Nickl graduated in Architecture at the ETH Zurich. During his three-year research period in Singapore, he managed urban development projects in Singapore, Malaysia and Indonesia. In early 2019, he joined the Board of Nickl & Partner Architekten AG. He is also Managing Director of Nickl & Partner Architects Asia LTD and Nickl & Partner Architekten Schweiz AG. A further focus of his work lies in the development of mobile and modular buildings in the health sector.

IV

Responses to global crises

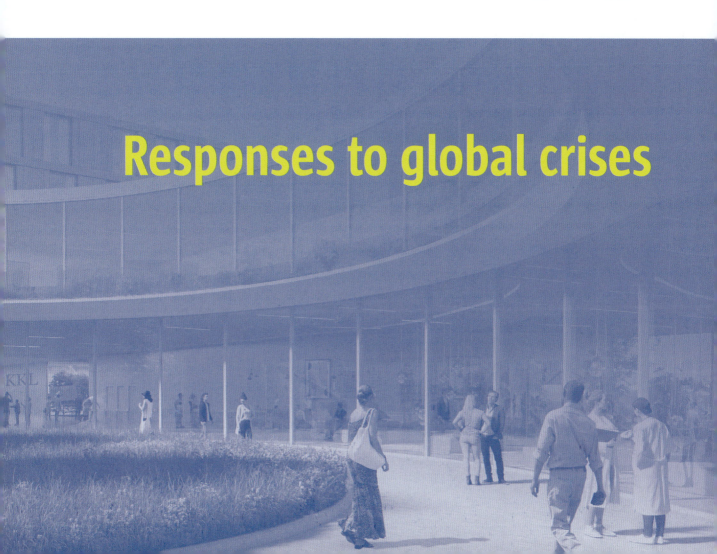

VII

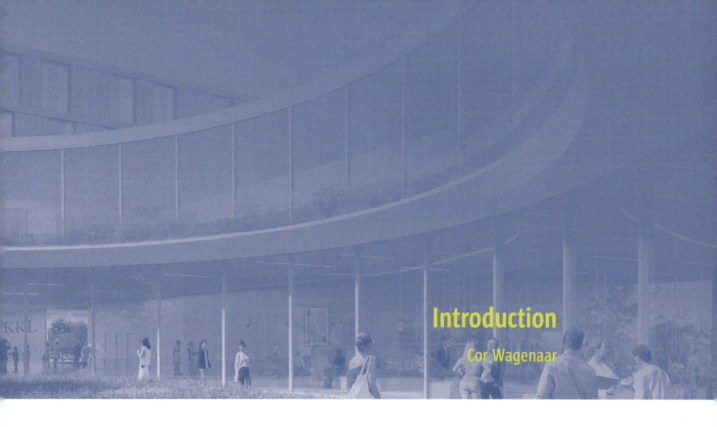

Introduction

Cor Wagenaar

One week before most of Europe went into lockdown, in March 2020, ENAH organised its eighth conference. We were just in time, but everybody felt that something was in the air, and it wasn't good. We were at the threshold of a period of global crises, and all of them had an impact on health. Two years later, in March 2022, our worst fears had become reality. This new reality framed our ninth conference. How can we deal with these crises? What can we do? We, architects, policy makers, technicians, consultants and forward-looking historians? Can we do anything? The sessions have taught us that we can. We have to try to make ourselves, our health care systems and our health care buildings more resilient.

Crises are nothing new. There have always been global crises. Covid has kept us busy for the last two years. When I entered the field of health care architecture, quite some time ago that is, medical doctors found it interesting to let us in on a little secret of theirs. One day, they said, a contagious disease will appear, and it will make the Spanish flu, which was the most devastating pandemic of modern times so far, look like only a minor thing. They seemed to enjoy sharing this piece of information with us. Apparently, it endowed them with the prestige that comes with knowing things hardly anybody else knows. A killer virus is on its way. It cannot be stopped.

Of course, nothing happened. Until, all of a sudden and out of the blue, Covid fell upon us. In the beginning we all thought that it was just another hoax—but it wasn't. Nor was it the killer virus that the medical doctors had warned us about. It was bad enough, but *im Großen und Ganzen* we got away with it very well. Public health is all about statistics, and statistically we could cope with this one. Personal tragedies also count, of course, but in public health they don't count for much. In the end, COVID-19 was nothing but a test run. What if the killer virus visits us? Maybe it is already flying above our heads—apparently, we have a severe case of bird flu that could develop into something else. We don't know. What did we learn? How can we prepare?

Pandemics are spectacular. The invisible, global health crises, however, are a lot worse. Air pollution kills ten million people every year. The WHO qualifies unhealthy lifestyles as a pandemic. There is nothing spectacular about these global crises—but they probably kill many more people than Covid has done.

One week before we happily came together in the Akademie der Künste for our ninth conference, another global crisis with a huge negative impact on health and mental health—the war in Ukraine—began. War is a permanent health crisis, as it directly impacts those involved in the conflict, but also causes feelings of uncertainty and maybe even fear all over the world. Wars have been going on all over the planet for decades—global peace is probably an illusion, but most wars never make the news. This one does. How can we address the consequences? What can we do?

Global crises are not exceptions, they are the rule. This final session, however, is not meant to be sad and downcast. Not at all. No matter how *unheimlich* the world has become, we need to be optimistic. And we will be. The three lectures that conclude this seminar address different ways to become more resilient in times of crisis.

The first theme focuses on the need for experts in this field to cooperate and create a field of equal opportunity and access to the expertise we need to address the many crises we are facing. Luca Fontana is an environmental toxicologist as well as an epidemiologist, and an expert in outbreak prevention, preparedness and response. He has first-hand experience with many infectious diseases. Michele di Marco is a scholar who combines knowledge of the planned environment with a passion for sharing knowledge. He sees knowledge sharing on an equitable basis as a fundamental human right. Both played a key role in founding Téchne, the World Health Organization's Technical Science for Health Network. Within the framework of the WHO, Téchne breaks new ground. It is the first branch that focuses on non-medical strategies to prevent diseases and promote health. One of the fields that helps to achieve this is architectural and urban planning. These impact health in many ways; after addressing issues of hygiene, pollution, housing and stress, the frontline has moved to the way our environment promotes (or frustrates) healthy lifestyles. Téchne incorporates research of scientific institutions, among them universities, which explore what technology can do make us more resilient in times of crisis.

Hannes Mayer is an internationally renowned specialist in the digitalisation of the design and construction processes in architecture. In his experiments with robotics, he breaks new ground. He also explores the use of artificial intelligence in architecture, and he will show some pretty amazing examples of his work with Gramazio Kohler. Will all these innovations lead to a giant leap forward in making our cities and our buildings more sustainable? And will the digital revolution really allow us to make non-standard, highly customised structures? Will it help us to meet future needs quickly and precisely, without environmental waste? And what can robots learn from the animal kingdom, from ants more specifically?

Edzard Schultz is principal architect and partner at Heinle, Wischer und Partner, and spokesman for the entire office. He teaches all over the world, and he has worked in crisis-ridden regions ranging from Venezuela to North or South Ossetia. He is fascinated by what he calls the "communicative synthesis in the architect's work." Schultz will show us how architecture has responded to the sudden need to build substantial numbers of intensive care units for Covid patients in less than no time—a formidable achievement and also an important learning experience. If we are under a lot

Introduction

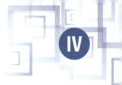

of pressure, we can manage to build these facilities. They are of a temporary nature—when we don't need them any longer, they can go. Here, the architect becomes a crisis manager and an expert in logistics.

Ideally, the three strategies to increase resilience can be combined in one coordinated effort. Technology that reaches beyond the limits of the medial world, the benefits of the latest technological innovations in the digital world, and the rapid response operation exemplified by the instant construction of intensive care units—they are the product of our new, crisis-ridden world. If these crises will not go away, these three examples may at least inspire a certain level of confidence: with the right tools, and above all the right mental attitude, we should be able to live with them, and hope to work our way to a somewhat happier world.

Prof. Dr. Cor Wagenaar

Groningen University/ENAH
Groningen
The Netherlands

Cor Wagenaar studied history at the University of Groningen. In 1993 he published a PhD thesis on the reconstruction of Rotterdam. He has participated in research projects sponsored by the Netherlands Organization for Scientific Research and the Royal Netherlands Academy of Arts and Sciences. In 2001 he joined the Institute of History of Art, Architecture and Urbanism at Delft University. Wagenaar has developed health care architecture as his second specialisation since the late 1990s, wrote numerous articles and books on the topic (among them *Hospitals. A Design Manual* in 2018, published in Chinese in 2023), and for a short time worked as a hospital consultant. In 2014, he was appointed Professor by special appointment at the University of Groningen, specialising in architecture, urbanism, and health. In 2016 he became full professor in the history and theory of architecture and urbanism, and head of the Expertise Center Architecture, Urbanism and Health. He chairs the scientific board of the Berlin based European Network Architecture for Health. Cor Wagenaar lives and works in Groningen and Berlin.

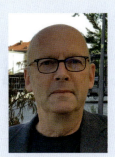

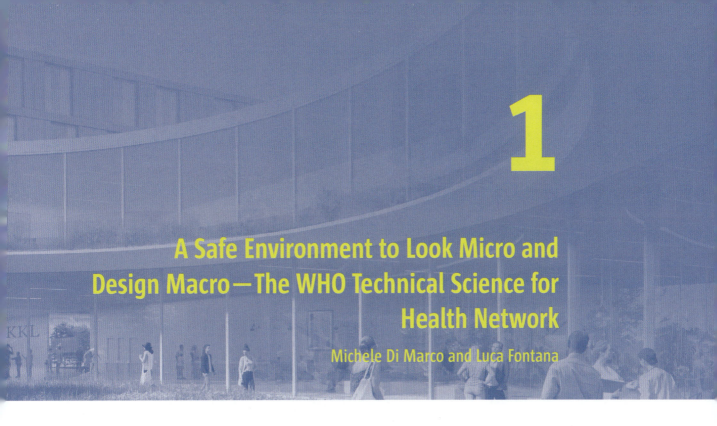

1

A Safe Environment to Look Micro and Design Macro — The WHO Technical Science for Health Network

Michele Di Marco and Luca Fontana

Diseases outbreaks and building environments are somehow bonded. They have had a long relationship: typhoid fever in the Athens of the fourth century which decimated its population by two thirds; Hansen's disease during the Middle Ages; the Black Death, a spread of the bubonic plague around the world that killed around a third of its population and caused the collapse of feudal systems and economic structures and redistributed the demographics charts in Europe (s. fig. 1); the seven cholera pandemics that prompted the creation of new sewage and water treatment systems all around the world; Spanish flu, SARS, and a long list of others. Starting from an historical perspective, this text focuses on the relationship between building environments and infectious diseases and the role that architects and engineers have in responding to epidemics.

Environmental and engineering measures play a key role for infection prevention and control in health care settings. The layout, flows, ventilation, wayfinding, finishing and materials, amongst others, contribute to reducing the risk of nosocomial infection while enabling

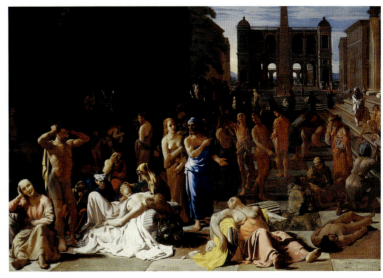

Fig. 1 Plague in an Ancient City, by Michael Sweerts, c. 1650 (available in Open Access via LACMA: https://collections.lacma.org/node/183358)

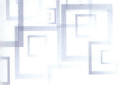

IV Responses to global crises

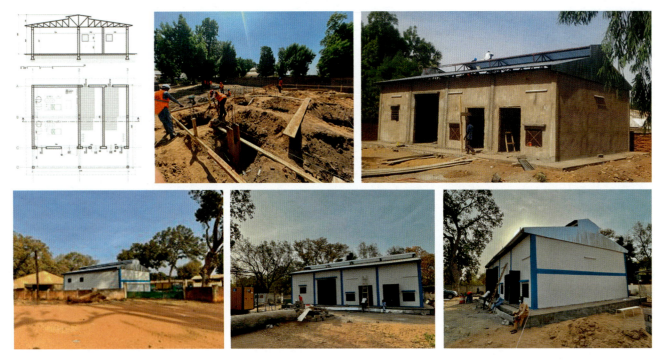

Fig. 2 Design of new health facilities

the provision of care in a safe and humanised manner. Drivers for the design and evidence for technical decisions come from different disciplines, highlighting an overlap between the medical, social and the building environment. Understanding pathogen-specific modes of transmission, care pathways and standards or care combined with setting-specific social and cultural aspects are essential for the development of more resilient and flexible health structures. Providing a common language and bridging the medical and building environment is the raison d'être of the WHO Technical Science for Health Network (Téchne).

In April 2020, in response to Member States' need for guidance and assistance in addressing technical aspects and structural challenges related to their COVID-19 response activities, WHO created Téchne, a multidisciplinary network of external technical institutions and universities which shares scientific knowledge and connects health, building and engineering disciplines. Téchne significantly contributed to the pandemic response on all levels, providing technical assistance to countries in all WHO regions on improving environmental and engineering controls to make health settings and structures safer for health workers and patients, and reduce the risk of hospital-acquired infections.

1 A Safe Environment to Look Micro and Design Macro – The WHO Technical Science for Health Network

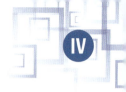

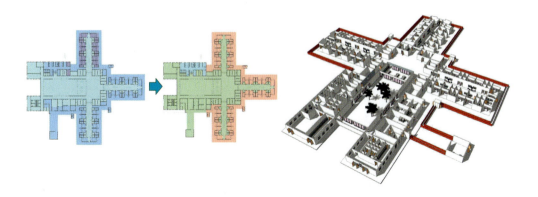

Fig. 3 Innovative structures bridging preparedness and response

Téchne support:
- design of new health facilities (s. fig. 2)
  - customised technical support to set up health facilities
  - screening, trauma centres, infectious diseases, oxygen plants and many more
- innovative structures bridging preparedness and response (s. fig. 3)
  - customised technical support to set up and run health facilities able to accommodate patients with different needs and risk status
- repurposing of existing facilities and surge plan development
  - the fastest and most efficient way to surge is to leverage existing resources
  - provide field and remote support to repurpose available structures into other services. i.e., repurposing of internal medicine into COVID-19 wards and repurposing of a basketball court into a quarantine facility
  - technical report for immediate implementation or as part of surge plan
- engineering and environmental controls for infectious diseases (s. fig. 4)
  - remote and field support to implement the most stringent structural requirements for infection, prevention and control
  - structures designed to enhance natural ventilation for airborne precaution and temperature control
  - patient and staff flows designed to enable the highest standard of care while ensuring safe and humanised care
- structural assessment, essential items, cost and HR estimation
  - technical support to assess structure and its functionalities including essential items availability and forecast, set up and running costs, and HR estimation
- trainings for infectious diseases treatment centre set-up, management and decommission (s. tab. 1)
- engineers, architects and WASH expert deployments
- national capacity building through international knowledge sharing

IV Responses to global crises

Fig. 4 Engineering and environmental controls for infectious disease

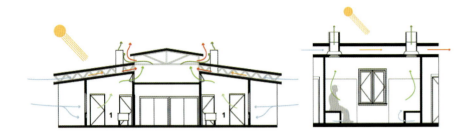

Tab. 1 Multidisciplinary training package and simulation exercise to enable rapid and effective response

Innovative Care Environments	Optimised Supportive Care for EVD	EBOV-specific Therapeutics
■ not just an *isolation* unit but a *treatment* facility centred around patients, families and the community ■ a place where patients can receive safe and effective care	■ oxygen and diagnostics systematic assessment and reassessment ■ hemodynamic resuscitation prevention and management of complications	■ proven in hallmark randomised clinical trial (PALM), there are two new molecules available to care for patients with EVD: Inmazeb (REGN-EB3), Ansuvimab (mAB114, Ebanga)

In less than three years, Téchne has responded to technical requests from thirty-five countries, contributed to the publication of three sets of guidelines and, through webinars and online workshops, advised forty-five countries on SARI, Ebola and Cholera facility design. It has also been involved in multidisciplinary research connecting health, building and engineering disciplines.

Téchne envisions the creation of safer, healthier, fairer and more sustainable health and care systems, settings and structures through integrated multidisciplinary community-based and informed approaches to problem solving. Téchne's mission is to facilitate access for Member States to the highest level of scientific knowledge available, to support in the technical aspects related to health emergencies preparedness and response.

The COVID-19 pandemic is an evolving global concern that impacts all countries in the world. At the same time, countries and communities continue to experience other disease outbreaks, humanitarian crises and natural disasters, impacting the lives of millions of people on an ongoing and regular basis.

Therefore, it is vital to reinforce and sustain national capacities to manage any emergency. The plan for the next five years is to have at least one Téchne member focal point in each of the 194 WHO member states. In this way, the Ministry of Health in each country can rely not only on the support of a trained national institution but also on the entire Téchne network. For more information about the WHO Téchne contact techne@who.int or visit the webpage www.who.int/groups/techne.

1 A Safe Environment to Look Micro and Design Macro — The WHO Technical Science for Health Network

Michele Di Marco

World Health Organisation
Division of Emergency Response
Geneva
Switzerland

Michele Di Marco is an architect and disaster risk reduction specialist with several years of experience in the humanitarian and development sector. Di Marco lectures at several universities on the topics of architecture, human rights, emergency response and disaster risk reduction. He is part of the founding team behind Téchne, the World Health Organization Technical Science for Health Network, where, in addition to working on engineering control for infectious diseases, he coordinates the Téchne members operations and activities.

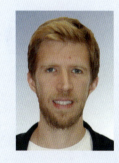

Luca Fontana

World Health Organisation
Division of Emergency Response
Geneva
Switzerland

Luca Fontana is an environmental toxicologist and epidemiologist and a WASH/IPC specialist, with comprehensive knowledge and extensive experience in outbreak prevention, preparedness and response. Fontana specialises in haemorrhagic fevers and has several years of field experience in Ebola outbreak responses. He also has notable experience with cholera, plague and other infectious diseases. Fontana has been working with Médecins Sans Frontières for more than six years and has been working with the WHO as WASH/IPC for highly infectious pathogens since February 2019.

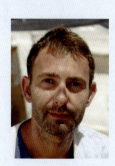

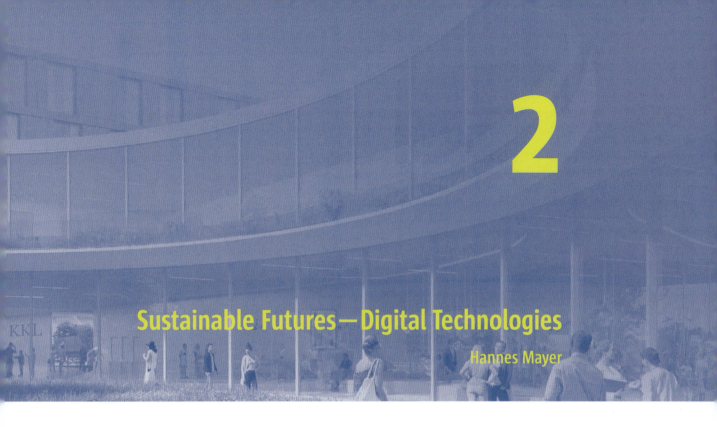

2

Sustainable Futures — Digital Technologies

Hannes Mayer

Since 2005, we have been researching how digital technologies transform architecture and, in doing so, what advantages they can bring for society.

Today, we face numerous crises, which challenge us on multiple levels. This means that incorporating new technologies into architecture is not simply about propelling the hype of innovation, but about utilising these new technologies in order to address the challenges we are facing in the building sector, such as material consumption, emissions and shortage of labour. This text is going to present a selection of projects that we have realised at the Chair of Architecture and Digital Fabrication—Gramazio Kohler Research—at ETH Zurich, to illustrate possible pathways towards solutions.

We designed and built the roof for the Arc-Tec-Lab, home to our institute and research lab. It covers a paradigmatic research environment and gives a distinctive atmosphere to this large open space. It is a load-bearing timber structure consisting of 168 timber frame trusses, each of unique geometry and internal composition. Almost 50,000 timber slats of three different cross-sections make up the trusses, which span up to twelve metres (s. fig. 1). Differentiating the cross-sections meant reducing material to focus it where it is needed. The slats, all similar but not identical due to their changing angles, are held together with approximately one million nails.

So, how do you design, manage and fabricate such complexity? The solution is an integrative design and fabrication approach that combines the knowledge of designers, engineers and those tasked with fabricating it in an iterative rather than a sequential process. The model is improved and optimised collaboratively, until the fabrication data can be sent directly to the machines for production by a portal robot and a numerically controlled circular saw. The portal robot cuts the pieces and builds up the 168 individual trusses layer by layer. An algorithm is used to calculate the exact position of each nail, and the portal robot connects the slats with an

IV Responses to global crises

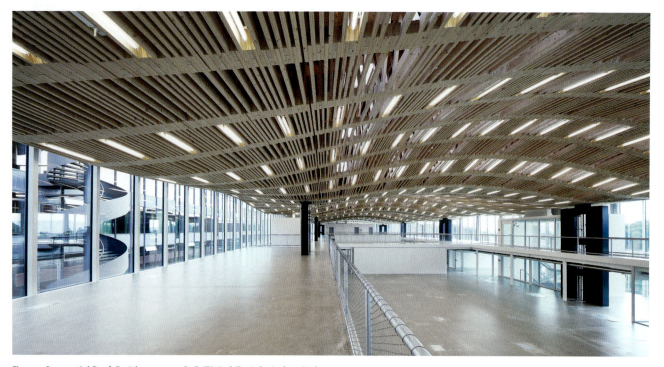

Fig. 1   Sequential Roof, Zurich, 2010–2016; © ITA Arch-Tec-Lab, Andrea Diglas

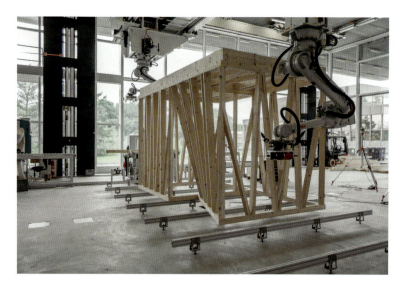

Fig. 2   Spatial Timber Assemblies, Zurich, 2016–2018; © Gramazio Kohler Research, ETH Zürich

integrated nail gun according to this digital data. At the end of the process, the result is visually checked against the digital model by the carpenter, who has acquired a new set of skills and tools to work with. The fabricated trusses are all similar but follow different curvatures while adhering to the same governing rules and procedures. Here, the modern understanding of architecture as a set of rigid standards gives way to rules that produce variations.

The same integrative method can be applied to three-dimensional timber frame modules. Starting from an initial typology—a spatial arrangement of lines—all information necessary for the fabrication process down to the individual screw is subsequently added in the digital 3D model. In the robotic fabrication lab, the modules can then be assembled by collaborating robots and a single carpenter. Each module is again unique but follows the same principles.

The Spatial Timber Assemblies project continues our research into building with timber, looking at the additive built-up of complex structures from simple elements (s. fig. 2). The modules designed and fabricated during the Spatial Timber Assemblies research project constitute the upper two stories of the DFAB HOUSE, an inhabitable research demonstrator developed by ETH Zurich and the National Centre for Competence in Research Digital Fabrication for Empa, the Swiss Materials Science and Technology institute in Dübendorf, near Zurich.

Another approach to integrating digital technologies into the building process is augmented reality. Instead of relying on a robotic arm for spatial manipulations, digital guidance is added to human dexterity. Using three wooden elements as an example, this technology can be easily explained (s. fig. 3). The system recognises the 3D shape of these pieces from digital images, which are inputs into the system by a camera. It then indicates where the carpenter must place the (next) piece of brick or wood by displaying a wireframe augmented onto the captured reality. For the production, the carpenters only need a specific camera, a laptop and a screen—on which they see the production steps displayed and receive all information for building the walls.

Such an approach provides sufficiently exact and intuitive guidance to the craftsman, eradicating the need for measuring angles and distances by hand. Working together with carpenters and the ETH spin-off Incon.ai, developers of the augmented reality app, we demonstrated the power of such a system with the realisation of an acoustic wall for the canteen of a large engineering firm in Zurich. The walls are composed of 8,500 identical wooden blocks of square cross-section with two angular cuts,

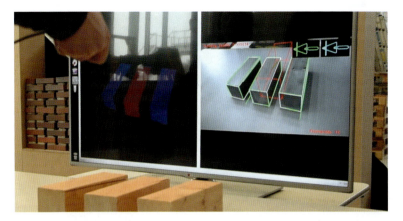

Fig. 3   Augmented Acoustics, preliminary study © Gramazio Kohler Research, ETH Zürich

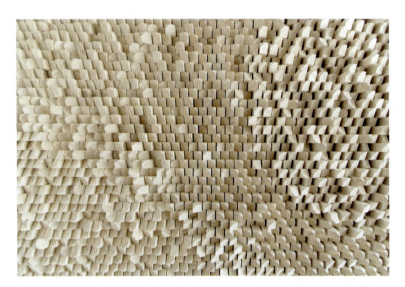

Fig. 4   Augmented Acoustics Detail, Esslingen, 2019; © Gramazio Kohler Research, ETH Zürich

which were then shifted horizontally and rotated by 90° (s. fig. 4 and 5).

Beyond geometries and form, digital technologies enable us to address various dimensions of architecture. They allow us, for example, to integrate acoustics, which is very im-

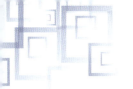

IV Responses to global crises

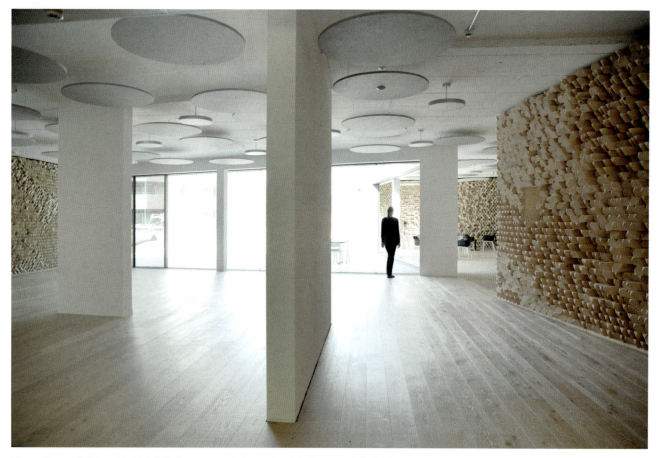

Fig. 5   Augmented Acoustics Detail, Esslingen, 2019; © Gramazio Kohler Research, ETH Zürich

portant for our well-being. Despite its importance, this is often overlooked or addressed at late stage. In the case of the acoustic wall, the design was programmed for an ideal degree of acoustic diffusion, and it also controlled the gaps between blocks for additional ventilation.

With the help of these new technologies, a new aesthetic and complex architectural language is created. Whether robotics or augmented reality, digital tools in architecture and construction allow humans to become smarter through computation, as they bring constantly evolving knowledge together from various fields. Digital production technologies help to materialise these informed designs, deploying newly found knowledge for a profession that is, by default, a complex field.

The following two projects emerged from a need to address the problems conventional building practices produce. Construction consumes an incredible amount of material and contributes to a huge amount of CO_2 emissions.

We can either improve the performance of existing methods, or think more radically about how construction can be reinvented by combining natural materials with digital technologies. For the Clay Rotunda at the SE MusicLab in Bern, our goal was to establish a cradle-to-cradle approach, which means that all the used material can be fully returned to its original state and re-used.

Instead of firing bricks at high temperatures, which results in high emissions, we extruded cylinders and brought them to the site as "soft bricks." Our mobile robotic platform was then used to perform the simplest operation a robot can do. It picked and placed each cylinder according to the digital model, pushing the material in a certain direction at a specific angle, which compressed each cylinder to about 30 % of its original height, resulting in the construction of a wall with a unique cobble-like appearance. One by one, the robot built the slender circular and undulating wall without any support or formwork. There is no magic involved here. It is just clay, sand, silt, and water, without any additives or chemicals (s. fig. 6 and 7). The key is the combination of digital control and the understanding of the behaviour of the material. In this way, a five-metre-tall structure with a diameter of twelve metres was built from 30,000 soft bricks, which, in the future, could simply be returned to the pit and made into new bricks.

The Rock Print Pavilion at the Gewerbemuseum in Winterthur, Zurich, involves a surprising transfer from science into practice. In this project we used gravel (crushed porphyry), commonly used as track ballast, and ordinary string. Our hypothesis was that using these two materials, we could make the aggregates interlock under compressive force, a phenomenon known as jamming. The research team developed a robotic process for laying the string in a circular pattern and for depositing small por-

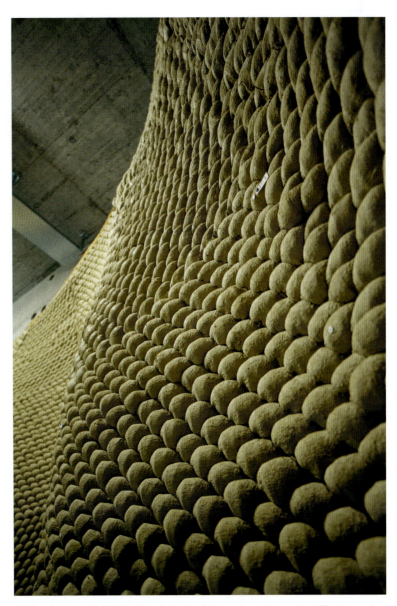

Fig. 6 Clay Rotunda Detail, SE MusicLab, Bern, 2020–2021; © Gramazio Kohler Research ETH Zürich

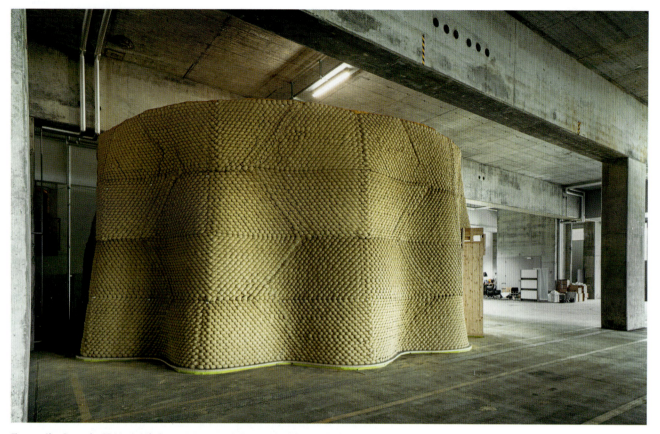

Fig. 7   Clay Rotunda, SE Music Lab, Bern, 2020-2021; © Gramazio Kohler Research ETH Zürich

tions of gravel. This allows for stable structures, built layer by layer, alternating between string and gravel (s. fig. 8).

In front of the Gewerbemuseum, we built a pavilion open to the public every day. Over forty tonnes of material were processed by a single robot, turning loose material into a stable structure of columns that cluster and turn into walls. A steel roof adds weight for the structure to jam and protects it from the weather. With digital control and robotic precision, a building is aggregated from loose material without any formwork or support. No waste is produced in this process. The building method only temporarily binds material. Once the building is no longer needed, the string can be pulled and wound back onto the spool. The gravel is thereby released, the building turns back into a heap and the process of turning a heap into architecture can start again.

Even though it may be difficult to imagine using these methods for the realisation of a hospital, the examples show what is possible today. With digital technologies in architecture, we can work on a more sustainable future for a "healthy" architecture and planet, and actively contribute to tackling the various crises that construction faces today.

2 Sustainable Futures — Digital Technologies

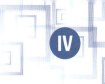

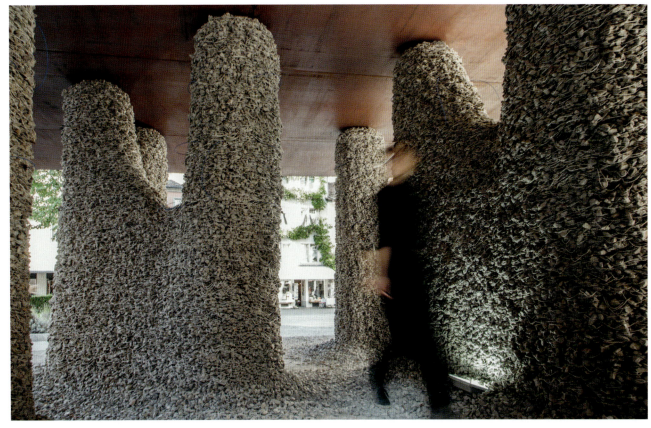

Fig. 8 Gewerbemuseum — Hello, Robot, Winterthur, 2018; © Gramazio Kohler Research, ETH Zurich, Martin Rusenov

Hannes Mayer

ETH Zürich
Gramazio Kohler Research
Zurich
Switzerland

Hannes Mayer is an international expert on digital transformation in architecture, and realises projects worldwide at the interface of science and architectural practice. At ETH Zurich, as a senior researcher with Gramazio Kohler Research (Chair of Architecture and Digital Fabrication), he led a pioneering research group for robotics and digital technologies in architecture for many years. Based on his research, he curated exhibitions on the digital future of building in cities such as San Francisco, New York, Milan, Venice, Tokyo and Zurich, and realised large-scale architectural installations, for the Centre Pompidou, V&A Dundee and Istituto Svizzero in Rome. He is the author of *How to Build a House*, about the DFAB HOUSE, the world's first inhabitable building created by robots, as well as editor of the magazine *manege für architektur*.

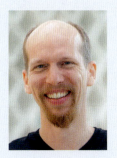

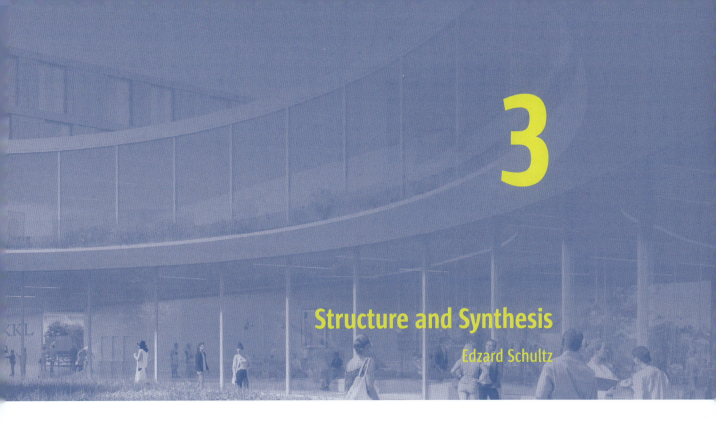

3

Structure and Synthesis

Edzard Schultz

Introduction

Health care buildings around the world are facing similar challenges in increasing patient acuities and, at the other spectrum of care, in rising volumes of ambulatory treatments. In turn, patient satisfaction and the patient experience continue to be key strategic drivers, as hospitals search for the right mix of standardisation and individual design to create a human-centred environment, which links the architecture to the specific site and its spatial references.

A modular design with standardised rooms is essential for high-tech areas of medical development, where industrial and scientific developments in medical technologies and procedures forces an ongoing and rapid change. Moving towards a modular structural program (which is composed of a handful of spatial modules, s. fig. 1), as an element of facility development, has incredible potential to facilitate the design and construction of the building (s. fig. 2).

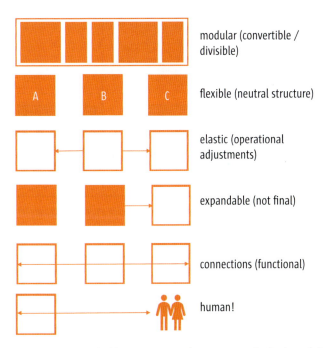

Fig. 1 Elasticity in buildung structures is the prerequisite for "enduring" the permanent change in medicine

IV Responses to global crises

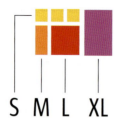

Modules	S 8 m²	M 16 m²	L 32 m²	XL 48+ m²
Rooms, areas, units (examples)	Workroom (small), restrooms, storage etc.	Examination, treatment, office, workroom (large), staff room etc.	Patient room, nurses station, conference room, work equipment etc.	Operation room, X-ray, MRI, CT, physiotherapy etc.
Vertical circulation	Elevator		Stairs	
MEP	Yes	Yes	No	No

Fig. 2   The spatial configuration of a hospital can be reduced to a few basic types (modules)

This data tool, along with generative design techniques, allows analysis and visualisation of design options based on varied data input. It examines flows of traffic within and between different departments before the planning stage is reached, and thus helps to optimise different layouts of the hospital in early design phase.

Example 1: Corona Treatment Centre Jafféstraße, Berlin

From the basic evaluation to the commissioning of a building project, there are nine service phases, which often stretch over several years. This was however not the case with the Corona

3 Structure and Synthesis

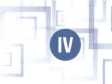

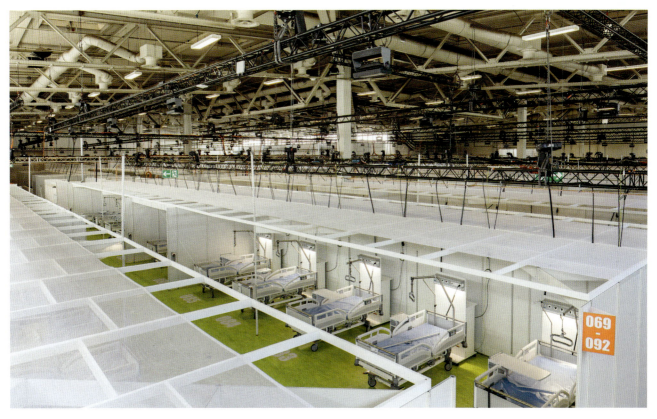

Fig. 3 The Corona Treatment Centre at the Berlin exhibition grounds was planned and realised within a few weeks. © Konstantin Börner, Nordsonne Identity

Treatment Centre, which was built within a few weeks on the Berlin exhibition grounds to relieve the hospitals in the event of a renewed increase in the number of infections (s. fig. 3). Where planning processes otherwise often run rather linearly, this rapid yet no less complex project required a high degree of simultaneity and dynamism. This unusual pace for construction projects was also accompanied by almost unique conditions and requirements for which there had been no precedent before; a completely new situation that called for flexible solutions.

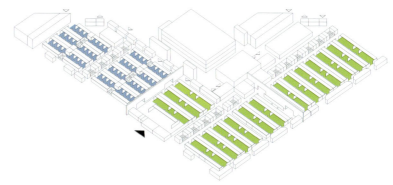

Fig. 4 The Corona Treatment Centre at the Berlin exhibition grounds, Hall 26, is divided into a general care area with 16 clusters of 24 beds each (green) and a respiratory care area with 7 clusters of 16 beds each (blue)

IV Responses to global crises

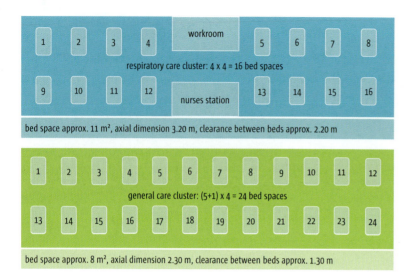

Fig. 5   A general care cluster is subdivided into 24 bed spaces, while the respiratory care cluster accommodates 16 bed spaces

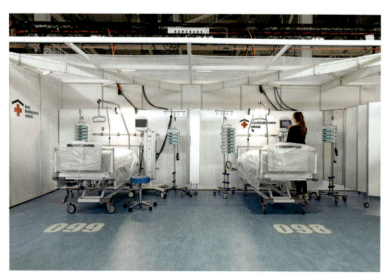

Fig. 6   111 respiratory care spaces were constructed in Hall 26 C, which were designated with the blue linoleum flooring. © Christian von Polentz/transitfoto.de

The Context

At the beginning of May 2020, Berlin is looking back on a now six-week-long exceptional situation triggered by the coronavirus pandemic. All over the world, health and supply systems are reaching their limits, and the fear of an overload of infrastructures is also growing in Germany. To prevent a bottleneck, the Berlin Senate decides to build an emergency treatment centre to create additional capacity for admitting corona patients. The Berlin Exhibition Centre makes two of its halls available and heinlewischer is chosen as the architecture firm to carry out the project (s. fig. 4).

The Concept

The architecture of an exhibition hall, if it is to be transformed into a hospital, brings with it both disadvantages and advantages. The sheer size of the space is both at the same time—the challenge of creating rooms within the space that meet the high standards of hygiene during a pandemic, and the opportunity to develop scalable structures that can flexibly adapt to the demands of the constantly changing situation.

Units with 16 to 24 bed spaces each are created in so-called clusters, whose mobile equipment can be adaptively adjusted to the individual medical and nursing requirements (s. fig. 5). The modular clusters also function as a blueprint for use in other locations. Thus, heinlewischer were also commissioned with the planning of an emergency treatment centre in Cologne, which also utilised the cluster structure and was further developed according to the specific requirements of the new location.

The Architecture

The construction of an emergency treatment centre is primarily about time and precision. In the face of these two imperatives of functional

3 Structure and Synthesis

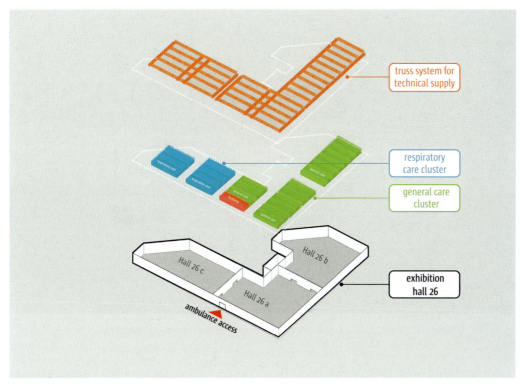

Fig. 7 The layout of the treatment centre is based on modular clusters with 16–24 beds and a central service zone. The oxygen lines for each bed space as well as the electrical and data technology supply are provided via cross beams, so called traverses, suspended from above.

rationality, the purely aesthetic form inevitably takes a back seat creating space for an unusual beauty of purpose that adapts to the special dimensions of an exhibition hall architecture.

To ensure good orientation within this exhibition hall, which covers a total of 11,690 square metres, a special wayfinding system was developed, whose large-scale elements can be recognised even from a great distance (s. fig. 6). Another special feature derived from the conditions of the exhibition hall architecture was the idea of routing all installations necessary for the building services via trusses. Thus, the lines required for the medical systems, ventilation and sanitary facilities are brought to the respective clusters from above via the trusses,

so that maximum construction freedom was maintained below (s. fig. 7). This construction method, typical for the trade fair and event sector, allows for a high degree of flexibility and also ensured that the ambitious deadline targets were met.

All systems were successively developed and continuously evaluated. Not only were the special requirements of the project itself an absolute novelty, but also the availability of information at the beginning of the construction phase. There was neither an overview of the project requirements in terms of rooms, functions and equipment, nor was there a detailed room programme. Everything that is usually determined in advance jointly by engineers, architects and

IV   Responses to global crises

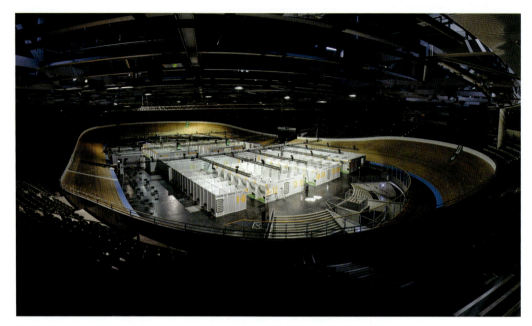

Fig. 8   Vaccination Centre at the Velodrom cycling centre, Berlin. © Konstantin Börner, Nordsonne Identity

clients had to be developed for this project while construction was already underway elsewhere—a sprint whose end is an emergency treatment centre that no one hopes to need at some point.

Example 2: Corona Vaccination Centres, Berlin

With the aim of vaccinating up to 400,000 people against the Corona virus in a first phase, temporary vaccination centres were set up at 6 locations throughout the city (s. fig. 8 and 9). Even though very different building typologies were converted for the vaccination centres from an indoor cycling track to a former airport they utilised the same modular system in their construction, which flexibly adapted to the local conditions. The uniform structure enabled rapid realisation in just a few weeks.

A wayfinding and colour system supports orientation in the vaccination centres. Thus, the important points of the vaccination process—registration, general education and the vaccination streets themselves—are marked by the guiding colour green. The wayfinding is supported by trilingual signage and pictograms. As all vaccination centres are located in large indoor spaces with little daylight, bright colours, such as a strong yellow-orange and a light green, were chosen for the elements of the wayfinding system.

Conclusion

With the modular structure of the clusters and the technical access via the trusses, a general blueprint on how to cope with such tasks in the future was developed. The Corona Treatment Centre has been done in a short time and it is adaptable for other places. In this respect, the most important finding of this project is actually its repeatability. We are optimally equipped and have good reason to be hopeful.

3 Structure and Synthesis

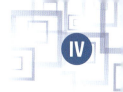

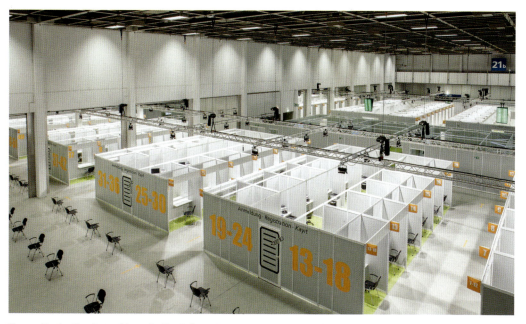

Fig. 9 Vaccination Centre Messe Berlin, Hall 21. © Konstantin Börner, Nordsonne Identity

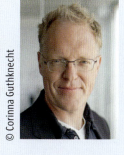

Edzard Schultz

heinlewischer Architekten
Berlin

Edzard Schultz is a principal architect and partner of heinlewischer and spokesman for the entire office. He studied architecture at the TU Berlin. To this day, he is also involved in teaching and research, for example at Clemson University South Carolina (USA) Architecture + Health. He is a member of the "AKG – Architekten für Krankenhausbau und Gesundheitswesen" and is active in the DIN committee. His work covers the broad spectrum of complex building tasks, primarily buildings for health, with a holistic approach from master planning through competitions and realisations to evaluation. He is especially interested in the structural and communicative synthesis in the architect's work.

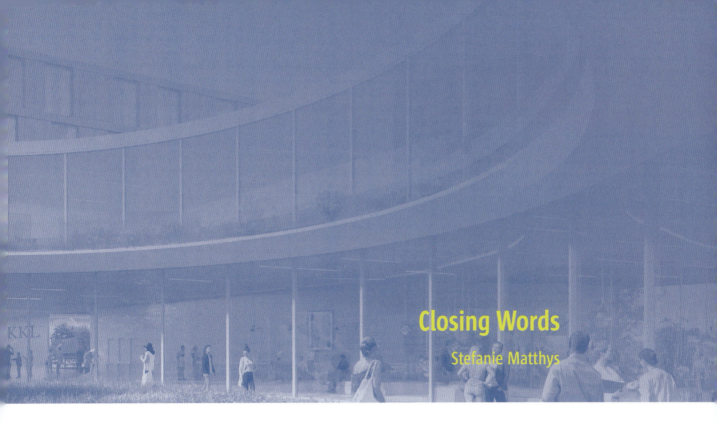

Closing Words

Stefanie Matthys

Fast & flexible—the ability to react quickly to unforeseen events and adapt flexibly to the challenges that the health care system will pose to its buildings in the future: this was the thematic thread running through the contributions compiled in this volume. They illustrate the deep uncertainty that the global COVID-19 crisis has brought to the health care sector. Above all, however, they shed light on the huge potential we are currently seeing in response to this challenge.

The four sections of the book present pioneering new architectural concepts that rethink building for the health care sector, such as the iconic "Hospital of the Future" by OMA, the floating hospital presented by Magnus Nickl or the Paris "Care Machine" by Brunet Saunier and Renzo Piano Building Workshop. There are also more experimental approaches, such as the master's thesis "Circle of Health"—a group of specialised community care centres on Berlin's S-Bahn ring—or the futuristic-looking fabrication techniques for a future in which buildings are generated with the support of robotics and AI.

The authors made it clear that the search for new, revolutionary forms of construction, planning tools and architectural concepts does not stem from the desire of an architect driven by weariness to do something "new", no matter what. Rather, the contributions from health care management and health care system research made it clear that these new concepts are a necessity. A necessity in a health care system that cannot help but reform itself due to cost pressure, inefficiency and staff shortages on the one hand and an unprecedented surge in innovation on the other. The report by Carolina Lohfert Praetorius and Henrik Praetorius on Danish hospital reform illustrates that this can be done in an organised manner and with measurable benefits. The fact that similar reform movements in Germany are not yet a done deal is clear today—two years after the conclusion of the conference whose contributions are collected here—in light of the heated discussi-

Closing Words

ons surrounding German hospital reform. They also make us realise that health care cannot be designed on the drawing board alone. Logically calculated scenarios for efficient, interconnected and quality-focussed care must form the basis of the reform, but the population's concerns about losing "their" local hospitals must also be addressed by offering convincing alternatives.

These alternative services will undoubtedly move in the direction of digitally connected "health care ecosystems" that combine home care and hospital care, as described by Nirit Pilosof, Eivor Oborn and Michael Barrett. It is now up to the planners—architects, urban planners, designers and engineers—to translate these new concepts into spaces that provide people with a sense of safety and security in these new, flexible and fast-evolving health care environments.

The European Network Architecture for Health (ENAH) hopes to make a contribution to this goal by bringing together experts from the architectural and medical world. This would not be possible without the support of partners from industry and the private sector, whom we would like to take this opportunity to thank very much.

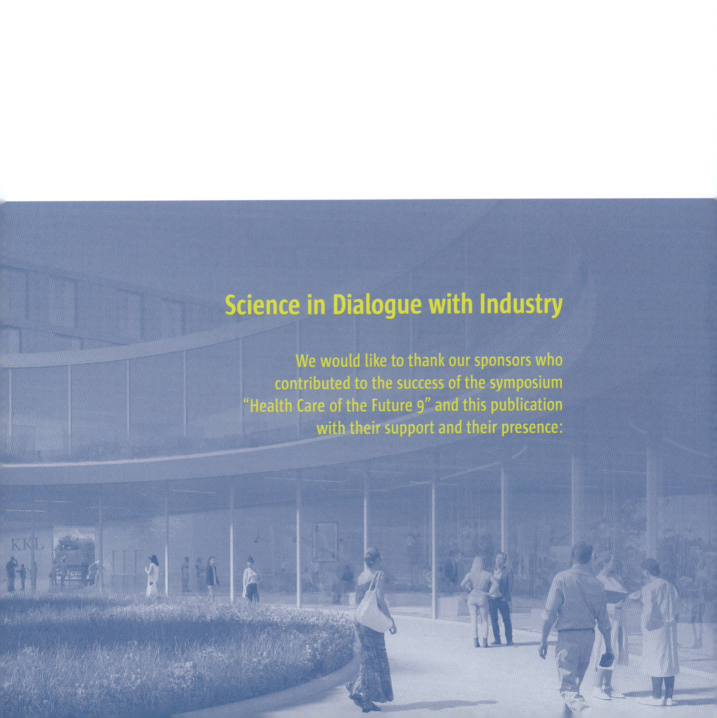

Science in Dialogue with Industry

We would like to thank our sponsors who
contributed to the success of the symposium
"Health Care of the Future 9" and this publication
with their support and their presence:

Science in Dialogue with Industry

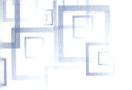
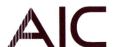

AIC is an international and independent insurance broker for the real estate industry with focus on major planning- and real estate risks, the design of multi-risk covers for major asset risks like building portfolios or healthcare building projects. Since 1998, multilingual contract specialists and lawyers accompany the interests of all AIC clients from the initial contact through the organisation of an insurance program until the settlement of claims. In our four locations nationwide (Berlin, Hamburg, Cologne and Munich) we employ highly qualified personnel for individual insurance solutions in the construction business. Our many years of experience regarding the insurance for general planners and leading architects in the hospital construction sector, helps both builders and planners to recognise risks and to guarantee a resilient coverage! In 2008 AIC Global Solutions GmbH was founded as a competent support and extension of the extensive range of services for all the special requirements beyond national borders. To continue the internationalisation process, AIC Swiss AG was founded in Zurich in February 2020. By using modern technologies as well as our own software and product developments, we ensure short processing times while providing valuable and transparent insurance solutions. Customer service is part of the mission statement of AIC.

| www.aic-international.de

The future of construction.
You have to love challenges if you want to shape the future of construction. For instance, cutting construction time down by half while maintaining the same high quality. Or turnkey handover on a specific date. Or fixed costs with subsequent building flexibility. From planning and production to assembly and operation.

As a module construction company and market leader for medical buildings, that is what Cadolto stands for. We also build offices and educational buildings, laboratories and cleanrooms, apartment buildings and hotels as well as data centres and telecommunication facilities. Permanent or temporary, for purchase or for rent.

We manufacture in our factory, regardless of the weather, under constant quality controls. With a maximum prefabrication level of up to 90%. This distinguishes Cadolto from virtually all of its competitors. With the experience of 770 projects executed worldwide, about 300 specialists from all trades, in two German factories and with 130 years of tradition.

Our modules leave the factory fully equipped. Including complete medical, laboratory and building technology, as well as washrooms, lighting, permanently installed furniture, etc. The constructors remain flexible: Additions, remodelling and dismantling, moving an entire building—everything is possible. And all with a high level of sustainability: no emissions at the construction site, 80% less truck traffic, reusability and 100% recyclable materials.

| www.cadolto.com

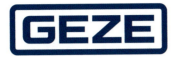

Since 1863, GEZE has been operating as a successful, global family business offering products, system solutions and services for doors and windows.

GEZE networks involve everyone in all the phases of the building life cycle and achieve outstanding results with thorough industry and specialist expertise. Together with its customers, GEZE joins projects at an early stage and provides long-term support to drive forward building development. GEZE offers modern, innovative door and window technology that makes buildings more liveable. Stable and yet dynamic, GEZE helps shape new trends, developments, and markets.

Over 3,154 people work for GEZE worldwide, with production locations at the headquarters in Leonberg, China, Serbia, and Turkey. With 37 subsidiaries all over the world, the company stays close to its customers and offers excellent service on site.

GEZE employs around 1,200 people at its main site in Leonberg. This is the where our international headquarters are located, including development, manufacturing, distribution and administration. GEZE has six branch offices in Germany.

www.geze.de

Science in Dialogue with Industry

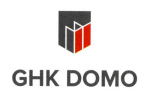

The company GHK DOMO GmbH develops, produces and markets system components for medical facilities worldwide. The design of holistic solu-tions, the use of high-quality materials and state-of-the-art manufacturing techniques lead to complete solutions for the highest demands, which are used in hospitals, clean rooms and laboratories.

The product range includes tailor-made operating room systems as well as door systems as revolving door and sliding door systems in modular construction. With many years of experience, GHK DOMO supplies and installs systems for operating rooms, cupboard systems, partitions and changing rooms. Ready-made sanitary cells, washstands, handrail systems for medical applications are manufactured both as standardised products and as individual room solutions.

GHK DOMO GmbH stands for material and processing quality and for the practical, professional execution on site. In addition to customer and service orientation, we specifically focus on the long-term functional reliability of our products, reliable availability and needs-based solutions.

Trespa Toplab Vertical is used for wall cladding in the operating room and functional furniture in critical areas. With this compact material, there is an advantage in terms of versatile colouring options and flexible processing. On the other hand, Trespa Toplab Vertical with its special EBC surface has excellent chemical resistance and does not promote the growth of bacteria.

www.ghk-domo.de
www.trespa.com

Science in Dialogue with Industry

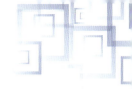
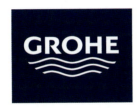

GROHE is a leading global brand for complete bathroom solutions and kitchen fittings and has a total of over 7,000 employees in 150 countries—2,600 of them are based in Germany. Since 2014 GROHE has been part of the strong brand portfolio of the Japanese manufacturer of pioneering water and housing products LIXIL. In order to offer "Pure Freude an Wasser", every GROHE product is based on the brand values of quality, technology, design and sustainability. Renowned highlights such as GROHE Eurosmart or the GROHE thermostat series as well as groundbreaking innovations such as the GROHE Blue water system underline the brand's profound expertise. Focused on customer needs, GROHE thus creates intelligent, life-enhancing and sustainable product solutions that offer relevant added value, and bear the "Made in Germany" seal of quality: R&D and design are firmly anchored as an integrated process in Germany. GROHE takes its corporate responsibility very seriously and focuses on a resource-saving value chain. Since April 2020, the sanitary brand has been producing CO_2-neutral (includes CO_2 compensation projects) worldwide. GROHE has also set itself the goal of using plastic-free product packaging by 2021.

In the past ten years alone, more than 490 design and innovation awards as well as several sustainability awards confirmed GROHE's success. GROHE was the first in its industry to win the CSR Award of the German Federal Government and the German Sustainability Award 2021 in the categories "Resources" and "Design." As part of the sustainability and climate campaign "50 Sustainability & Climate Leaders", GROHE is also driving sustainable transformation.

| www.green.grohe.com

LIXIL (TSE Code 5938) makes pioneering water and housing products that solve everyday, real-life challenges, making better homes a reality for everyone, everywhere. Drawing on our Japanese heritage, we create world-leading technology and innovate to make high quality products that transform homes. The special thing about LIXIL is how we do this; through meaningful design, an entrepreneurial spirit, a dedication to improving accessibility for all and responsible business growth. Our approach comes to life through industry leading brands, including INAX, GROHE, American Standard and TOSTEM. Approximately 55,000 colleagues operating in more than 150 countries are proud to make products that touch the lives of more than a billion people every day.

| www.lixil.com

Science in Dialogue with Industry

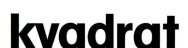 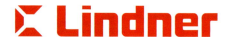

Kvadrat develops high quality modern textiles and textile-related products. Our products reflect a commitment to colour and simplicity, along with the desire to develop textiles based on innovation and experimentation in design. Our fabrics are for you to innovate, to design and to create.

www.kvadrat.de

The Lindner Group is Europe's leading supplier, manufacturer and service provider for the interior fit-out, building envelopes and insulation. We are a true family business with a deep understanding for "Building New Solutions", the development and implementation of custom-fit and advanced yet flexible project solutions and room concepts. We do this in all service phases: from the initial idea, through the design and planning process, to the execution and assembly as well as the subsequent service—for new buildings, renovation and refurbishment.

Over the last decades, we have developed into a technically strong and reliable partner with a solid economic basis. With sustainable concepts such as Cradle to Cradle Certified®, low-emission products and well-thought-out room concepts, we want to create Add.Vantage—for your project, for people and for the environment. As service provider and employer, we put people first, which is what the customer notices too: We enjoy our work, are confident in what we do and are proud of what we can achieve.

With a workforce of more than 7,500, we operate numerous production facilities and subsidiary companies in more than 20 countries from our main offices in Arnstorf, Germany.

www.Lindner-Group.com

Science in Dialogue with Industry

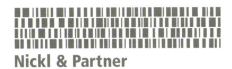

Nickl & Partner

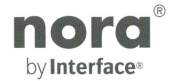

Our internationally active office devotes itself to the planning and construction of buildings in the health care, research and social housing sectors, as well as town planning for the private and public sectors.

Our goal is to create modern buildings which positively boost working and living spaces. To us, architecture means understanding and ordering things whilst focusing upon people. To a large extent, the designs of Nickl & Partner are based upon the actions and needs of people who work, live and receive health care there. Their wellbeing in addition to the perfection, functional interplay of flexible spatial designs and exciting materials is our key concern when performing our work.

We rank among the leading architect's offices in Germany in the fields of medical facilities, clinics and research institutes. Our specialist expertise in the fields of technology and building materials is very extensive and our innovative concepts have proved themselves over a period of more than 3 decades.

Since the founding of Nickl & Partner in 1979, the team has grown to approximately 180 members. National and international clients from all areas of healthcare, research and urban development have entrusted us with planning and implementation.

| www.nickl-partner.com

nora systems is a leading global manufacturer of rubber floorcoverings for commercial applications and part of the Interface Inc. The robust and high-performance nora® rubber floorcoverings have been produced in Germany since 1950. In health and care facilities, they are characterised by high comfort, cost-effectiveness, and optimal hygiene. nora® floorcoverings are not only easy to clean, but also completely disinfectable, making them suitable for use in high-risk areas where regular surface disinfection is required. Thanks to their extremely resistant surface, they are highly wear-resistant, and their flawless appearance is maintained for many years. With their broad, harmonious colour spectrum, nora® floorcoverings create a feel-good ambience in all rooms. The rubber floorings are free of PVC, phthalate plasticisers, and do not contain any polymers containing chlorine. All nora® standard products have been awarded the eco-label "The Blue Angel."

| www.nora.com

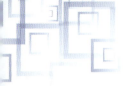

Science in Dialogue with Industry

SCHÜCO

70 years of Schüco—System solutions for windows, doors and façades. Based in Bielefeld, the Schüco Group develops and sells system solutions for windows, doors and façades. With 5,650 employees worldwide, the company strives to be the industry leader in terms of technology and service, both now and in the future. In addition to innovative products for residential and commercial buildings, the building envelope specialist offers consultation and digital solutions for all phases of a building project—from the initial idea through to design, fabrication and installation. Schüco works with 10,000 fabricators and 30,000 architectural practices, as well as construction professionals who commission buildings around the world. Founded in 1951, the company is now active in more than 80 countries and achieved a turnover of 1,695 billion euros in 2020.

| www.schueco.com

Triagonal®

Triagonal is a leading design firm providing strategically anchored wayfinding strategies and design services globally. Decades of experience within the field and a great number of prestigious projects, awards and recognition have made Triagonal a trusted wayfinding partner, creating value for our clients, users and society. We are an interdisciplinary team of passionate professionals including graphic and industrial designers, engineers, strategists and anthropologists. All with creative experience and a user-centred approach to all phases of a project—from fieldwork and analysis, to concept development, implementation and evaluation. Our major areas of operation are complex environments like hospitals, airports and transportation hubs, as well as major cultural and educational institutions.

| www.triagonal.info

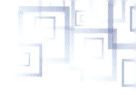

Thanks to our network partners

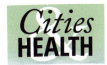 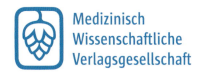

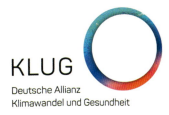

as well as our academic partner

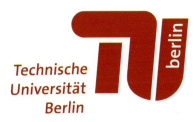